GREEN GUIDES

Running

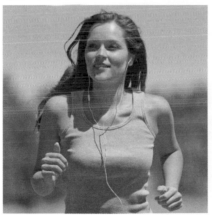

This is a **FLAME TREE** book
First published 2012

Publisher and Creative Director: Nick Wells
Senior Project Editor: Catherine Taylor
Copy Editor: Sonya Newland
Picture Research: Laura Bulbeck
Art Director: Mike Spender
Layout Design: Dave Jones
Digital Design and Production: Chris Herbert

Special thanks to Caitlin O'Connell, and to Magellan PR, Fitbrands and TCL Sports in addition to the companies listed below in the picture credits.

This edition first published 2012 by
FLAME TREE PUBLISHING
Crabtree Hall, Crabtree Lane
Fulham, London SW6 6TY
United Kingdom

www.flametreepublishing.com

Flame Tree Publishing is part of Flame Tree Publishing Ltd
© 2012 this edition Flame Tree Publishing Ltd

ISBN 978-0-85775-389-2

A CIP record for this book is available from the British Library upon request.

The following images are copyright © as follows: Clif Bar 153; Compressport (www.compressport.uk.com) 64, 89bl, 89br; Hammer Nutrition 152; Inov-8 52cl, 57t, 57b, 74tr, 94; Jelly Belly Candy Co (www.jellybelly-uk.com) 151t; Maraisthon 30r, 30bl; Newline (www.newlinesport.com) 65tl, 76tl, 76br, 80br, 81l, 81r, 82r, 83, 84bl, 87, 88bl, 92, 108; Newton Running UK 52tr, 55, 56b; www.2XUshop.co.uk 78, 90, 126. All other pictures are courtesy of Shutterstock.com and © the following photographers: CandyBox Images 1 & 119; Val Thoermer 3 & 45 & 245, 14, 174; Gemenacom 4br & 33, 156; Supri Suharjoto 4l & 16, 185; Warren Goldswain 5l & 49; xc 5br & 62; AISPIX by Image Source 6l & 96, 41bl, 192bl, 201; Maridav 6br & 128, 8, 12, 28bl, 112, 122, 214; l i g h t p o e t 7tl & 180, 17, 29, 82l, 86 & 247; Richard Waters 7r & 215; fotohunter 9b & 54; Martin Novak 9t, 161bl, 234; Kovalev Sergey 10; Daniel Korzeniewski 11t, 50tl; Patrick Poendl 11br, 44tr; samotrebizan 13, 208; JHDT Stock Images LLC 15br; Yun Yulia 15tl; Kurhan 18, 99; jsimagedesign 19l, 207; Marin 19br; auremar 20tr, 135; Piotr Marcinski 21, 188; AdventureStock 2272 & 252, 229bl; Kzenon 23, 136tr, 138; mkrberlin 24tr; Tamara Kulikova 24b, 26l, 212; patrimonio designs limited 25, 39bl; wavebreakmedia ltd 26br, 133, 198br, 228bl, 240, 241r; Tyler Olson 27r, 46l, 155bl, 204br, 209br; Valua Vitaly 27; Stefan Schurr 32, 51tl, 75; Sue Robinson 34; jan kranendonk 35bl; Shawn Pecor 35tr & 253; July Flower 36; David Burrows 37tl, 124; Diego Cervo 37br, 202; Maxim Petrichuk 38; Anetlanda 39tl; Gorilla 39c, 88tr, 143; Demid Borodin 41tr; Rob Wilson 42, 182, 193; Gary Blakeley 43tr; Pete Saloutos 43bl; Chad Zuber 44bl, 228tr; Photoroller 46tr; Phase4Photography 48, 101, 176br; Mark Atkins 50br; Baronb 51r; Nomad_Soul 53& 246; roobootb 56t; EpicStockMedia 58; Christopher Edwin Nuzzaco 59tl, 187r; gosphotodesign 59br; Dan Thomas Brostrom 60; Arpi 63, 68, 69, 84tr, 171b; AM-STUDiO 65br, 158; Darren K. Fisher 66; Peter Weber 67, 79; Shestakoff 70; testing 71; Jiri Slama 73; Byron W.Moore 74bl; Losevsky Pavel 77; Blazej Lyjak 80tl, 170tr, 194tr, 221, 223r, 224 l; homydesign 85; Shane White 91, 206l; Vaidas Bucys 93; AVAVA 97, 118l; Dmitriy Shironosov 98; karen roach 100; Käfer photo 102; ArtmannWitte 103; Chris Curtis 104l; trevorb 104br; Natalia Siverina 105; holdeneye 106; WiML 107; Olena Zaskochenko 109; Coprid 110; nito 111; Maciej Oleksy 113; Ilona Baha 114; Richard Peterson 115br; Tompi 115t; maxstockphoto 116bl; Tatiana Volgutova 116t; niederhaus.g 117; Irina Nartova 118r; Aleksandr Markin 120, 142l; Brendan Howard 121br; Martel 121l; Daniel Wiedemann 123; klohka 125; Peter Bernik 129, 210; MartiniDry 130; FotoYakov 131tr; StockLite 131b; Elena Elisseeva 132br; LeventeGyori 132t; Lisa S. 134; Fotokostic 136b, 231tl; Denis Kuvaev 137tr; Walter G Arce 137br; David P. Lewis 139t; Stanislav Fridkin 139br; vera-g 140; EdBockStock 141r; Jeff Cleveland 141bl, 196l; Dan Bannister 142r; terekhov igor 144tr; Timothy Large 144bl; barbaradudzinska 145; Crisp 146cr; digieye 146br; Monkey Business Images 146tl, 165, 166tl, 171t, 187l, 194bl; gillmar 147bl; RusGri 147t; Igor Dutina 148r; margouillat photo 148bl; inxti 149bl; Oliver Hoffmann 149cr; stockstudios 149tr; fotohavran.eu 150; crazychris84 151bl; Gerald Bernard 154; Jackie Smithson 155tr; Charles Knox Photo 157&249; Galushko Sergey 159t; itsmejust 159br; pics721 160, 175; Richard Thornton 161tr, 184tl; Alex Hinds 162; koh sze kiat 163bl, 237tr, 238; Rob Stark 163tr; Juriah Mosin 164, 239l; T-Design 166br, 196r; Mammut Vision 167; Andresr 168tr; Deklofenak 168l; Elnur 169; Lein de Leon 170bl; Valeriy Lebedev 172; Jack Z Young 173tl; Nils Z 173br; tungtopgun 176tl; bikeriderlondon 177t; Stephen Mcsweeny 177b; Andreja Donko 178; Rena Schild 181; duoduo 183tl, 205; Ron Kloberdanz 183br, 209tl; Vasaleks 184br; Photobac 186; Africa Studio 189t; Kris Butler 189b, 203, 237bl; ostill 190; Michaelpuche 191; Freddy Eliasson 192r; Johanna Goodyear 195tr; Martin Lehmann 195bl; Frank Herzog 197& 250; Stephen Coburn 198tl; Rafal Olkis 199; David Fowler 200b; Suzanne Tucker 200t; Malyugin 204tl; Phoric 206r; Alain Lauga 211, 235; NotarYES 216; Kameel4u 217; Luis Santos 218br, 231br; Yuri Arcurs 218tl; Capifrutta 219l & 251; ESLINE 219r; ppart 220; Anneka 222, 226bl; Susan Montgomery 223bl; stefanolunardi 224r; carroteater 225tr; Mike Flippo 225bl; Roblan 226br; Bork 227; murat5234 229tr; Radu Razvan 230; Borzee 232; Irena Misevic 233; Galina Barskaya 236; Tatiana Popova 239br; Vladimir Jotov 241l; Graça Victoria 242.

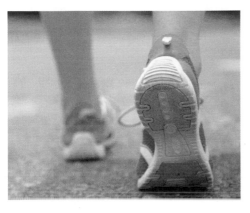

You may think that running starts with shoes, but in fact it starts with feet! This chapter explains how your foot type affects your running style, which in turn informs what type of footwear you should choose. This section will help you understand what to look for and what questions to ask when buying your running shoes. Our 'anatomy of a shoe' will help you jargon-bust before taking a closer look at the three main types of shoe – road, trail and 'barefoot'.

This chapter takes you through the 'big three' essentials – T-shirts, shorts and socks – before moving on to other items of clothing, including base layers, bras and jackets. There is also information on season-specific clothing and the additional apparel used for trail running. The subject of compression wear (those terrifying-looking super-tight leggings and tops) is demystified here too. Finally, this section discusses running sunglasses, and offers some no-nonsense advice on what to look for when selecting your shades.

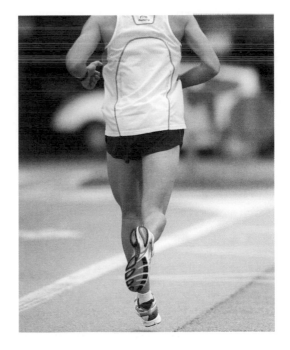

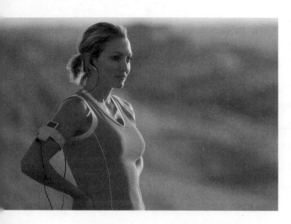

There are hundreds of running gadgets available – some vital for improving your running, others less so. When it comes to simply measuring your running distance, options vary from simple pedometers to expensive GPS sports watches. This chapter will help you weigh up the relative merits of the key gadgets, and highlights some of the new generation of smart-phone apps. Staying safe while running is of paramount importance, and safety gadgets such as reflectors and lights should be on your list of 'must-haves'.

Now it's time to get started. This chapter takes you through the basics of running health and sets the benchmarks for measuring progress. Safety, diet and the importance of good hydration are all explored, as are issues surrounding age, pregnancy and ill-health. This section also includes the standard structure of a run and the benefits of cross training. When you're good to go, you can start with one of our three basic running plans: general health and weight loss; improving stamina; and increasing your running speed.

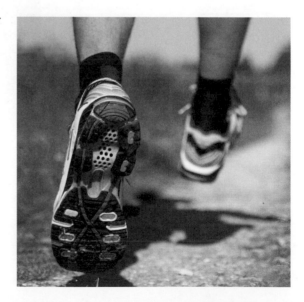

Training & Advanced Running 180

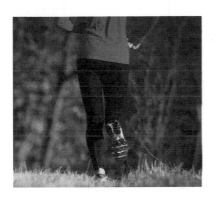

If you've followed the plans in the previous chapter – or are a more experienced runner already – this chapter helps you take your running further, looking at a range of exercises to improve your performance. It questions what *type* of runner you are and explores the world of running clubs, online networks and more. The four main race distances are covered in more detail here, along with suggestions for improving speed over 5k, full training plans for other distances, and essential race-day tips.

Troubleshooting 214

Beginning with some general injury advice – in particular the near-miraculous effects of ice packs – this chapter takes you through the world of running injuries, from heel bruises to back pain, with easy-to-follow guides to signs, symptoms and treatments. Of course, we hope you never have to make use of this chapter, but forewarned is forearmed and as your adventure into the world of running continues, you may find you have to treat the occasional blister!

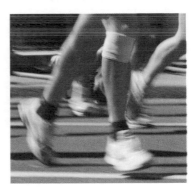

Checklists 244

Further Reading & Websites 252

Index 254

Foreword

If I was going to have one motto for my life it would be 'I run, therefore I am'. I have always been a runner, ever since I was capable of saying 'boots on, outdoors'. This love of running is an essential part of my make-up – and I wouldn't have it any other way.

Of course, I've had to come to terms with my own limitations as a runner (that I never made it to the Olympics will always be a source of disappointment to me) but it has made me realize that running isn't necessarily about being competitive. It's a sport that, with a little motivation, we can all enjoy.

There is no greater feeling than putting on your trainers, heading out the door and off the beaten track to be at one with nature; running delivers this time and time again. Running can be individual or it can be very sociable, with like-minded people drawn together by their love of this sport.

And in today's increasingly environmentally conscious society, running has just about the lowest carbon footprint of any sport. All you need is a decent pair of trainers, some basic kit and a willingness to be out in the open.

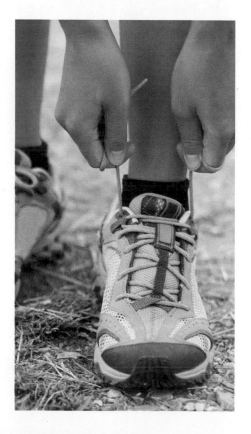

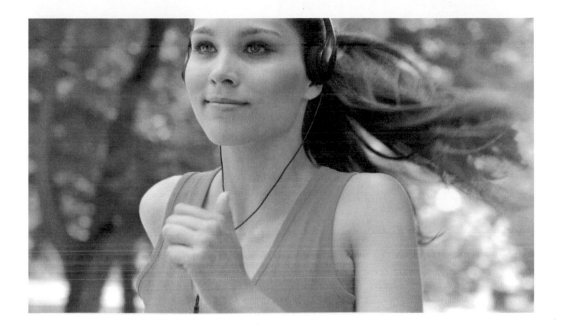

This message is at the heart of *Green Guides: Running*. This intelligently written and informative publication is packed full of advice for anyone new to running or individuals looking to improve. The fact that it also has the environment in mind is an added bonus.

If you've never run or simply need some advice to get you up and out the door, then this book could be the perfect answer. But don't just take my word for it. Read on and get an insight into just what a wonderful sport running is. Let *Running* help you discover the runner in you.

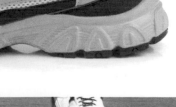

David Castle
Editor of
Running Fitness magazine

Introduction

Humans have always run. In ancient times, running could make the difference between going hungry and catching prey – or worse, becoming prey. Today's enthusiasm and motivation for running is less about life and death, but the point remains that running is perfectly natural. Learning to run – or, more accurately perhaps, re-learning to run – is not like learning to levitate or walk through walls. We were all born to do it.

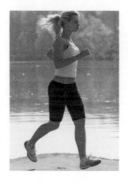

Explosion of Running

The modern obsession with running – certainly as a means of keeping fit – can be traced back to the 1970s, when the likes of America's Jim Fixx and New Zealand's Arthur Lydiard, among others, helped popularize it with the masses and kick-started something of a health revolution. Today, running is a global phenomenon, with thousands of converts taking to the streets and trails every year. Major cities in every part of the world stage mass-participation running events and festivals.

A Global Community

Being part of the running community is a wonderful opportunity. You will never be alone as a runner. Almost every town and village now has a running club and, if not, the internet provides the ultimate global running organization. Most runners are not only able but incredibly willing to share their knowledge and experience. Take part, share and learn.

Easy In

Put one foot in front of the other, then do it again. How easy could running be? Repeating that simple process over increased distances or with improved pace is all there is to it. Certainly you

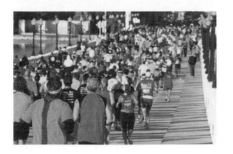

will need to learn some techniques, and understand how diet and general health play a role, but becoming a runner really couldn't be easier. The same is true of the kit and clothing required when you start out – shoes, shorts, socks, top ... and go. Shop around for some bargains (without skimping on the shoes!) and you could be ready to run for less than £100.

The Benefits of Running

The wealth of benefits running provides will be explored in the coming chapters, but the following list gives a good overview.

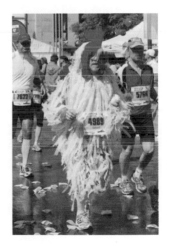

- **Feeling good**: Running is good for you. It really Is as simple as that – everything from your head to your heart will thank you for becoming a runner. It builds muscle, improves circulation, aids weight loss ... the list is endless.

- **Doing good**: Each year, runners raise millions for charities. The London Marathon, for example, is the largest annual fundraising event in the world!

- **De-stressing**: Few things clear the mind and de-stress the body better than a quick run.

- **Saving money**: Increasingly popular as a method of commuting, running can also save you a small fortune on gyms and exercise classes.

- **Proving a point**: Think you can't do it? Or been told by others that *they* think you can't? Prove yourself and others wrong – lace up your shoes and hit the streets. Self-belief is one of the most important things running will teach you.

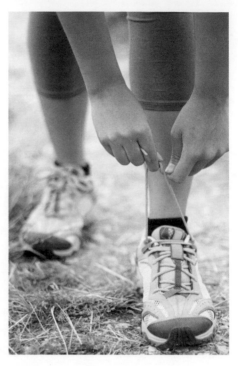

Being sociable: Meet like-minded people by joining a running club or connecting online with millions of runners worldwide – you'll be amazed how quickly your circle of running buddies grows.

Getting out: Treadmills are the rainy-weather resort for runners, but *real* running takes place outside. Enjoy the beautiful countryside or explore the back roads of cities. Get out and do it!

Exploring: Whether you're planning new routes, trailblazing adventurous runs or just wondering, 'Where does *that* road lead?', running is the perfect way to explore new areas or rediscover old ones.

Going further: If you find yourself hooked on entering races, you could find yourself enjoying previously unexplored corners of the country – maybe even the world.

Sheer joy: Few activities match the buzz of the 'runner's high'. Have fun!

Environmental: What could be more environmentally friendly than relying on nothing more than your own body to deliver all the above benefits? Running is the ultimate 'green' power!

You've probably already identified a reason or two from the list that match your motivation for buying this book. But if you still haven't made up your mind why you want to run – or even *if* you want to run – read on …

About This Guide

There is something for everyone in this book. Those taking their first tentative steps will be guided gently through the early days and, as confidence grows, on to the achievement of their first goals. Those looking for fresh challenges can follow the advice and training plans for their first half-marathon, or even full marathon. Even the most experienced runner will find the guides to shoes, clothing and injury invaluable.

You'll notice that throughout the book I avoid the words 'jog' and 'jogging'. This is personal preference – even if you are taking things at a slow pace, if you are not 'walking', you are 'running' – but whatever you call it, this book will help you achieve your potential. You will also notice the occasional repetition of advice – this is entirely intentional and meant to emphasize important information.

Feet First

Although running is a relatively inexpensive pastime, you will need to prepare yourself for a small initial outlay, and *nothing* is more important than shoes. The right shoes lead to comfortable, injury-free training and racing; the wrong shoes result in quite the opposite. Whether you are looking for shoes for road or trail (or indeed the 'barefoot' options), it is essential to have your feet professionally assessed and shoes fitted.

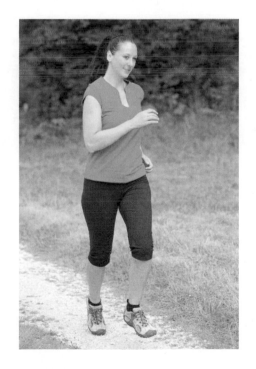

Kitting Up

We explore both the clothing basics – shorts, T-shirts, socks, etc. – along with a range of apparel likely to be useful once you extend your running or start to specialize (in off-road running, for example). Keeping costs down is important in these straitened times so choose wisely, particularly when it comes to additional running gadgets. Some of these can be immensely useful (and some even vital for safety), so understanding their value will help you prioritize.

Fit For Life

Taking a look at your general health and understanding just a little of the science behind running is a great place to begin. All this is covered in the 'Getting Started' chapter, along with the importance of water and food. Don't worry – it's not all mung beans.

Staying Safe

Safety when running is paramount – this cannot be stressed enough. Follow our common-sense advice, take a few simple precautions and you should enjoy years of trouble-free running.

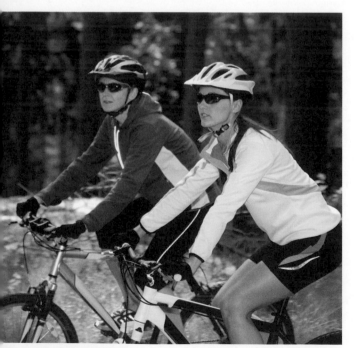

The Routine of Running

Every run you take should follow the same general pattern: warm up, run, cool down, stretch. Of course, we go into more detail on this in the book, as well as taking you through the benefits of cross training, such as cycling, swimming and yoga. Getting into a weekly routine, however pushed you are for time, can be easy and will help your running progression enormously.

Test Yourself

Time for a challenge? If weight loss is your goal (the second most common reason for taking up running, after 'general health'), there are three simple

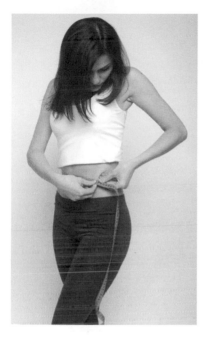

running plans to follow. The first is for general weight loss – and should always be followed in conjunction with a sensible diet – while the second and third plans will help you increase your distance and then your speed.

Going Further

If you've followed the advice in the Getting Started chapter, or are reading this as a more experienced runner, it might be time to step things up a little. The section on Training and Advanced Running discusses ways of improving your skills and eases you along the path towards a half-marathon or, perhaps the ultimate goal, the full 26.2-mile marathon. The key to successfully achieving these longer-term goals is small, incremental improvements. Never fear – you *can* do it!

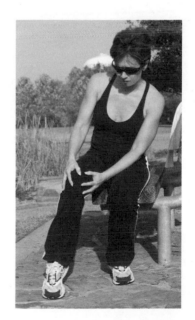

Feeling the Pain

Although running is undeniably good for your health, from time to time runners get injured. Knowing what is wrong and how to treat it is a vital skill; so is knowing when to seek a doctor's advice. Our guide to injuries is by no means exhaustive, but we cover the most common injuries and provide some simple, no-nonsense treatments. As you'll discover, the benefits of a good ice pack can never be underestimated!

Wherever your running takes you and whatever your goals in taking up this cheap, healthy, environmental and immensely enjoyable activity, have fun!

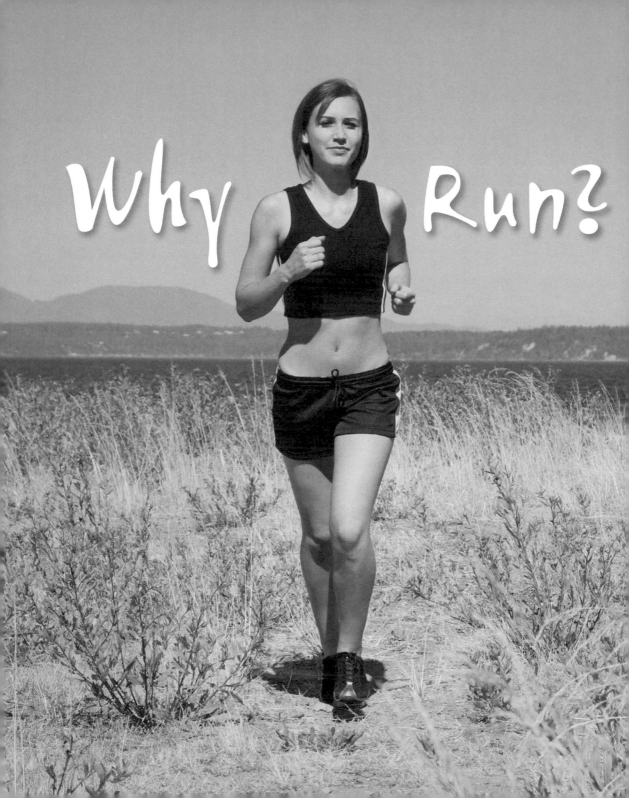

Why Run?

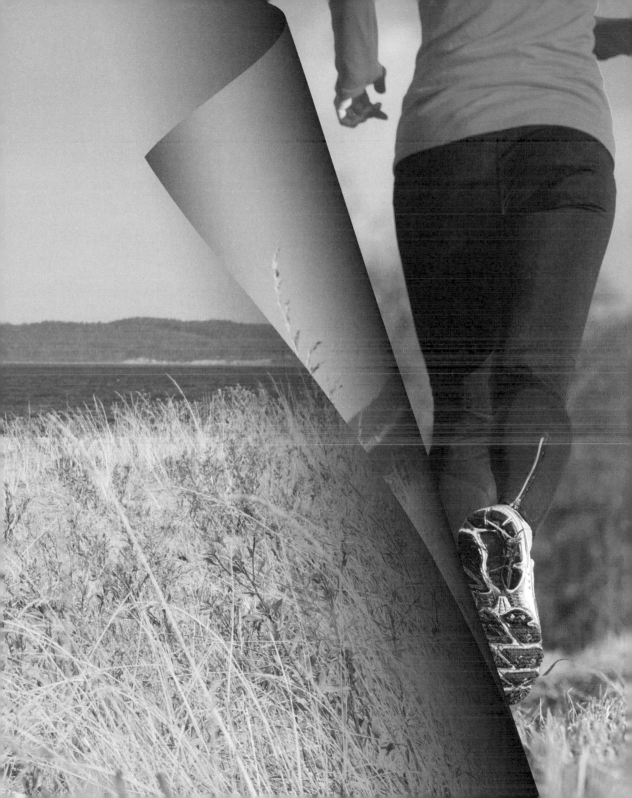

Getting Healthy

There are almost certainly as many reasons to run as there are runners. As it's unlikely that someone else is *making* you run, then taking to the streets is probably a self-motivated exercise. Perhaps it doesn't do to over-analyse your personal reasons for undertaking something that has so many obvious benefits, but health and weight loss are among the most common reasons for running.

A Boost for Your Body

Taking up running is *great* for you. Fact. Even accounting for some additional wear and tear to the body (being bad for the knees is largely a myth), the health benefits massively outweigh the occasional blister or aching muscle. Improved health is the number one reason for taking up running, and it is easy to see why.

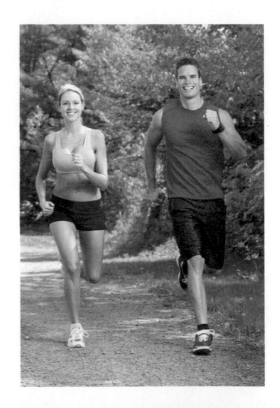

Be Inspired

'If you want to become the best runner you can be, start now. Don't spend the rest of your life wondering if you can do it.'
Priscilla Welch,
Olympian marathon runner

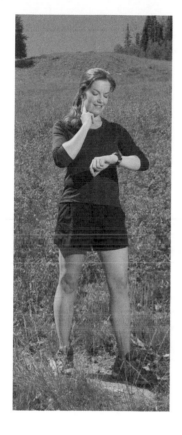

Healthy Heart

Scientific evidence has shown that running is one of the best forms of aerobic (oxygen-related) exercise for improving both heart and lung functions. It increases efficient circulation of blood through the body, not only during running but long-term, and is proven to help reduce the risk of a heart attack. The heart is a muscle and, in the same way that weightlifting increases the size of other muscles, running increases the size of the heart. A larger, more muscular heart pumps more blood per beat, resulting in a reduced heart rate – which is excellent news for your health.

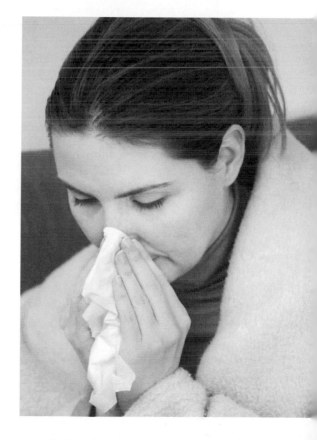

Self-defence

One of the 'hidden' health benefits of running is the boost it gives your immune system. Multiple studies have shown that exercise such as running three times a week can increase the circulation of macrophages (the white blood cells found in body tissue), which are an important part of your defence mechanisms. Research suggests that runners may be between 25 and 50 per cent less likely to contract a range of illnesses, including sinusitis, laryngitis and even the common cold.

Asthmatics Run Too!

It is astonishing to consider the range of conditions and illnesses with which it is not just *possible* to run, but is actually *beneficial*. Asthma is a prime example. Although this is a condition that affects the lungs, as long as certain precautions are taken there is no need for asthmatics to rule out running as a pastime, and many will find that their doctors encourage it. It is vital that the asthma is fully under control and that a doctor has been consulted – but beyond that, only a few simple steps are needed: always warm up and cool down to give the airways time to adjust; carry an inhaler at all times; avoid common triggers (atmospheric or pollen conditions); and stay alert to changes during the run.

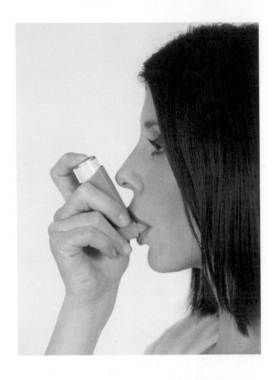

Weight Loss

In conjunction with a balanced diet – which broadly means watching your intake of saturated fats, sugars and junk food – running can be an excellent way to help lose weight. Dieting alone, with all the associated temptations, will take far longer to yield results than a sensible combination of running and healthy eating. Running at between 60 and 70 per cent of your maximum heart rate (*see* page 132) will burn the most calories, and with just a little practice this should be a perfectly comfortable 'zone' in which to run.

Stress Bust

If you favour exercising alone, then running provides excellent 'me time' in which to unwind and put problems into perspective. If, on the other hand, you prefer running with friends, then you will appreciate the group activity and companionship. Either way, running is an excellent way of busting stress. Science backs this up too – runners show reduced levels of adrenaline and cortisol (both stress hormones) and increased DHEA (dehydroepiandrosterone), which is thought to have a positive impact on stress. Best of all, running can be an instant cure to a moment of stress: shoes on and out the door ...

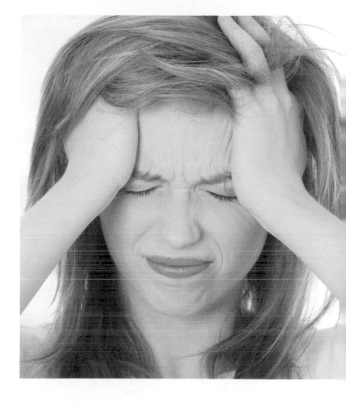

Look Good, Feel Good

Running gives you:

- **Lower blood pressure, reducing the risk of a stroke**
- **A strengthened immune system, resulting in fewer colds and respiratory infections**
- **A more 'sculpted' physique – increased muscle tone and reduced fat**
- **A strengthened heart, reducing the risk of a heart attack**
- **Reduced stress levels from lowered adrenaline and other stress hormones**
- **Improved lung capacity through better oxygen delivery**
- **Balanced cholesterol by increasing 'good' cholesterol and reducing 'bad' cholesterol**

Exploring Your World

With running comes an incredible sense of freedom and adventure, and there is no better way of exploiting this than exploring new areas, new routes – even new countries. As your running progresses, and your ability and confidence grow, you will begin to discover a whole new world.

Blaze a Trail

Although your first forays into running will probably be on familiar territory – a run around the block, your local park or city centre – there will come a time when you feel the need to explore a little further afield. Online running communities are an excellent place to start; with thousands of runners sharing their knowledge of routes and trails, you're sure to find something to suit.

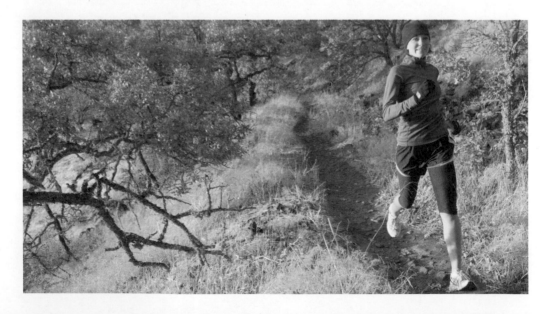

Beyond this, hours spent studying local maps and planning your own new routes is a joy in itself, and discovering a previously unexplored back road or cross-country trail brings a new dimension to your running.

Follow the Crowds

With races from 5k to marathons held all over the country, there is every reason to use your running as an excuse to explore those places you've always meant to visit, but never quite found the time. Taking the family or travelling with friends is a great way of combining a race or two with some sightseeing – and to remind yourself that travel in your home country should never be neglected for the glamour of a foreign holiday! Mass-participation runs usually offer a party atmosphere, and the main race event is invariably just a part of the wider attractions on offer, serving up the perfect balance of effort and reward.

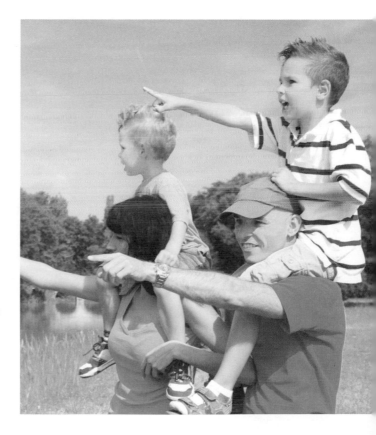

Globe Trot

The world is a big place and the world of running equally so. Think of a major global city and there will almost certainly be a race staged there. Many specialist tour operators cater for runners' needs, but if you want to look beyond the fully catered option, you can usually make your own arrangements to split race entry from travel plans. The majority of races offer their websites in a range of languages and most – with an eye to attracting foreign participants – are within easy reach of airports and other transport hubs.

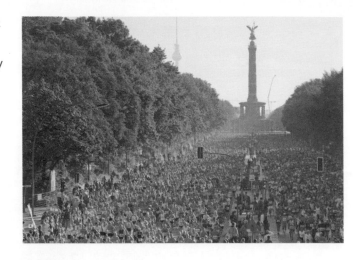

Plan Ahead

Taking your running kit with you on your regular holiday can be an excellent idea too. Not only is a run a great way of exploring your new surroundings, but it can also be a good ice-breaker, helping you to meet local runners eager to share their knowledge and local expertise. Maintaining your running routine on holiday will also go some way to offsetting the excesses of food and drink that can be involved!

Be Inspired

'No matter how many goals you have achieved, you must set your sights on a higher one.'
Jessica Savitch, broadcaster

Making a Difference

Every year, millions are raised by marathon runners for charities around the world. But you don't need to commit to anything as challenging as a full 26.2 miles to start making every stride count, and there is nothing more motivating than knowing that all your effort has such worthwhile results.

Choose Your Cause

With so many worthwhile causes to raise money for, picking a charity can seem almost as daunting as putting in the miles. In the first instance, it is important to choose a charity with which you have some connection or personal affinity. For example, many people run for medical charities that seek cures for diseases that have claimed the lives of loved ones. Having a genuine interest in a charity's work will provide extra motivation as well as help you talk passionately about it when fundraising.

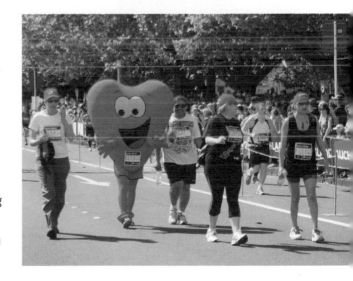

Get a Head Start

Many charities have guaranteed places (sometimes called 'bonds') at large races. You can apply for these in exchange for making a pledge to raise a minimum amount of sponsorship – a great way of gaining a place at otherwise hard-to-enter events. Also, check to see how much a charity can support *you* – many have excellent training plans and help forums to help you reach your goal.

The Keys to Running for Charity

Here are some of the main things to consider when planning a charity run.

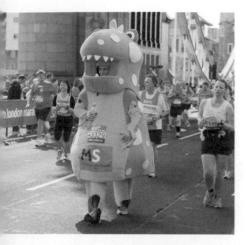

Be realistic: Make sure that both the race and fundraising goals are achievable, but ...

Make it unusual: Yes, a marathon is a challenge, but doing it dressed as a dinosaur is tougher!

Be passionate: Learn all you can about your chosen charity and talk about it with enthusiasm.

Mix it up: Add to the fund's target with cake sales, raffles and anything else that will add to the pot.

Get social: Social media sites such as Facebook and Twitter are an excellent way of getting your message out there.

Offline media: If your challenge is great enough or your story unusual enough, try getting the local newspaper or radio station interested.

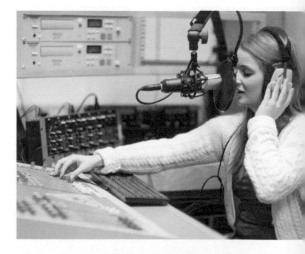

Tell everyone: The more people you tell, the more money you're going to raise.

Train sensibly: Follow your training plan, don't overdo it – and stay focused.

Social Running

Although you might take your first strides as a runner alone (possibly under the cover of dark), once you've found your confidence your social life is bound to benefit, as you make friends from around the world who share your passions. Even the most introverted runner can benefit from the wisdom of others, and a shared interest is always the right place to start a new friendship.

The Virtual World of Running

They might not seem like 'real' friends, but the internet is a world of unlimited information and potential when it comes to meeting like-minded individuals. Hundreds of forums and chat rooms are dedicated to running and, if you use the online running logs (where you can record your runs and set out your goals), you'll quickly find yourself a member of the global running community. Thousands of podcasts and videos are available on every aspect of running, and the more online running buddies you make, the more you will share and learn.

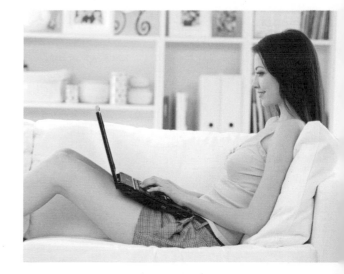

Top Tip
As with all internet use, be cautious about who you are talking to, and never reveal personal details or private information.

Real-world Running Mates

If the internet seems a little too impersonal, there are many opportunities to make friends out in the real world. Running clubs – a superb source of advice and information – often mix weekly training sessions with social activities, and whatever your level of ability you'll be welcomed and fully included. If you can't find a club, or at least one that suits you, consider starting one of your own.

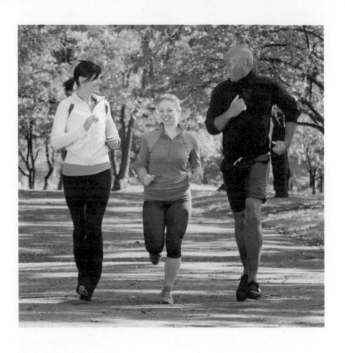

Familiar Faces

Even if clubs do not appeal, run the same route long enough and you'll begin to see the same familiar faces. You might soon find yourself running side by side and, hopefully, motivating one another.

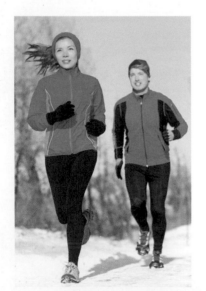

Take the Challenge

Growing your circle of running buddies is a sure-fire way of developing a little friendly competition. At first, this may just mean pushing yourself beyond your running comfort zone to increase the pace and keep up, but this can evolve into more ambitious challenges. There is no greater motivation to do well in a race than knowing your friend or partner is running it too!

Going Green

Running is pure 'green' power – just fuel your body and run. There are no emissions (at least not harmful ones!) and it leaves only a small carbon footprint, if you factor in the manufacture of your shoes and other running clothing.

Rush-hour Run

Running may not be quite the ideal environmental alternative to commuting that cycling can be, but a growing number of people are lacing up their shoes for the run to work. More and more companies are accommodating this trend by providing workplace showers and changing facilities. After all, a healthy workforce is a happy workforce.

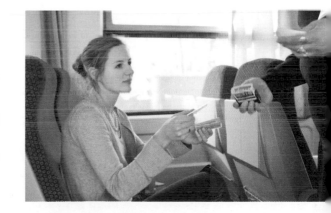

Get Fit, Save Money

Running to work is a great way of combining your favourite healthy pastime with the chance to save money on car bills or train fares. In the mornings, it will give you some thinking time to plan for the day ahead, and the run home is the ultimate way to de-stress and unwind.

Planning Your Commute

Your regular road running shoes and kit (or trail versions if your commute is cross-country) will serve you well for commuter running. The only additional item you need to consider is a running pack in which to carry a change of clothes. Do not be tempted to use a regular backpack – choose one specifically designed for the ergonomics of running (see page 126).

Racing Green

A growing number of environmentally aware races are appearing on the events calendar with each passing year. These 'green' races aim to drastically reduce waste, recycle wherever possible and encourage a fully sustainable approach to running.

Choosing Your Green Race

All major events should have a 'green' policy in place, but look out for races with a specific mandate

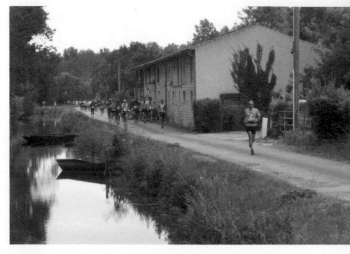

The Maraisthon is held in Coulon on the river Sèvre Niortaise.

such as the 'Maraisthon', held annually in the Marais Poitevin area of France. Along with the 26.2-mile challenge (promoted as the 'Green Marathon'), there is a 10k race that shares the same ethical approach, using entry fees to offset estimated environmental impacts, and even offering a finisher's medal in the form of an organic soap-on-a-rope. With the continued success of the Maraisthon, others are following in its footsteps.

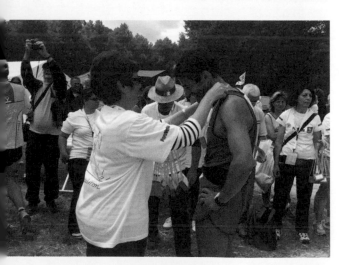

Soap-on-a-rope 'medals' are handed out at the Maraisthon.

Be Inspired

'I was 12 when I started and 34 before I achieved my dream; that should give people hope.'
Dame Kelly Holmes,
Olympic gold medallist

Checklist

- **Set your goals**: Even if your targets are initially unfocused – 'to get fit', for example – try to identify goals that will keep you motivated.

- **Explore**: Even the most familiar city or suburb takes on a new dimension once you start to run. Seek out the unusual routes.

- **Travel more**: Is there somewhere you've always wanted to visit? Chances are there will be a race or running event nearby.

- **Get involved**: Either online or off, form a club or get together with others with similar goals and running ambitions.

- **Off on holiday?** Pack your running shoes!

- **Stay safe**: Online security and safety is vital – keep alert.

- **Do it for charity**: What could be more motivating than raising money while you run? Signing up for an event that will push you to train harder too!

- **Get eco-friendly**: Seek out events that have a clearly defined environmental policy, or help your local race establish one.

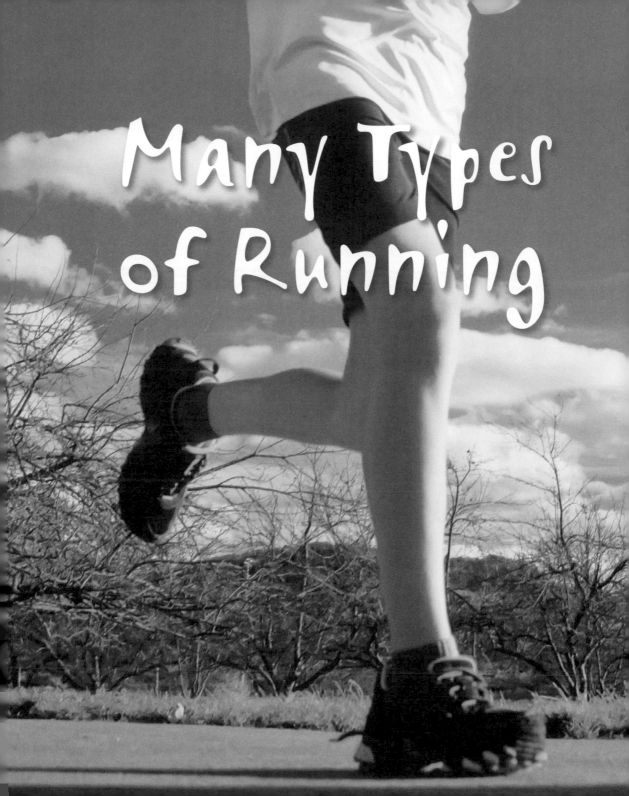

Many Types
of Running

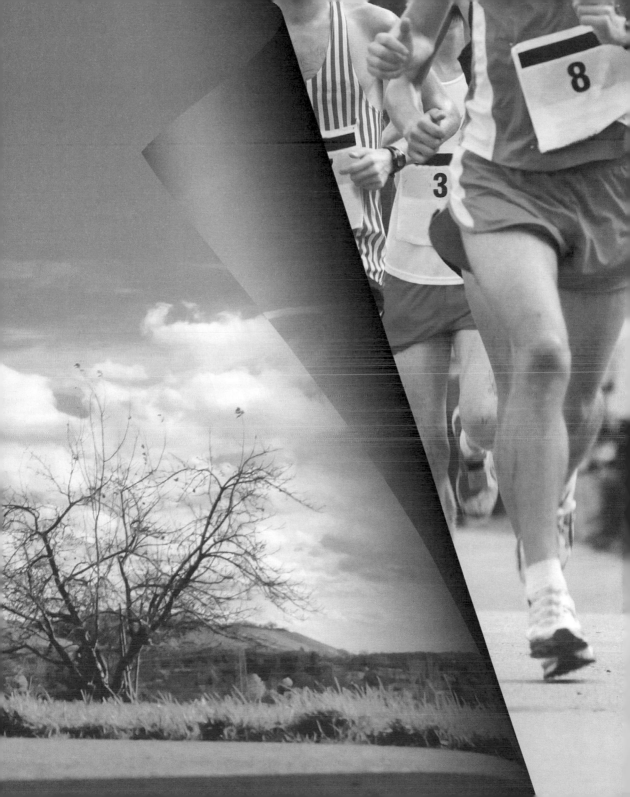

The Variety of Running

Running can broadly be divided into 'road running' and 'trail running' (or 'off-road running'), but factor in the many terrains and weather conditions – which can include mountain, woodland, footpath, mud, snow, city… to name just a few – and multiply this by the many *reasons* to run (health, social, global travel, etc.) and the combinations are almost endless.

Types of Organized Race

Once you are confident with your running, you will probably consider entering an organized event or race. Again, there are almost limitless combinations to choose from, including many easily achievable 'fun runs' (often involving fancy dress) and even lots of family events, which can include a range of distances with something to suit everyone.

Going the Distance

The most common distances for organized races are five km (always known as '5k'), 10 km (10k), 10 mile, half-marathon (13.1 miles) and marathon (26.2 miles). For most runners, the phrase 'inch by inch, life's a cinch; mile by mile, life's a trial' will apply – meaning that they will progress through these distances, conquering each in turn. Of course some runners may head straight for the marathon, but striving for a series of increasingly

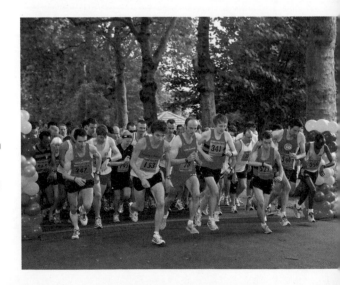

tougher challenges will allow you to build slowly and stay motivated. It's always good to have a new challenge on the horizon.

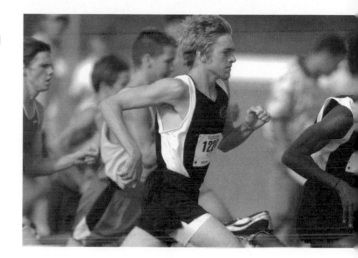

Be Inspired

'Success isn't how far you got, but the distance you travelled from where you started.'
Anonymous

Running Further

As incredible as it might sound, the marathon is not the final word when it comes to long-distance running – in many ways and for a growing number of runners, it is quite literally just the beginning. So-called 'ultra' events take place around the world, and these go far beyond the 26.2 miles of the *mere* marathon. These include 'entry-level' races of around 30 miles to extreme distances of 150 miles or more.

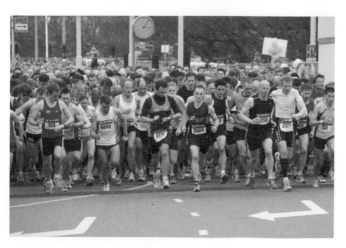

Just as most runners build up to their first 10k or half-marathon, competitors in extreme runs gradually increase their training and event distances – the only difference being that their starting point is likely to already be a marathon.

Road Running

For most new runners, their first experience will be road running – technically, and more safely, *pavement* running. Although there may be times when it is necessary to actually run in the road, even seemingly quiet country lanes can be hazardous and extreme care should be taken.

Simple Start

One of the things most people love about road running is that it involves simply stepping out of the front door. Your regular route cannot get more convenient than that, making it less likely that you will find an excuse *not* to go for that run.

Top Tip

Always be aware of cars reversing out of drives when running on pavements. This is a frequent danger for runners.

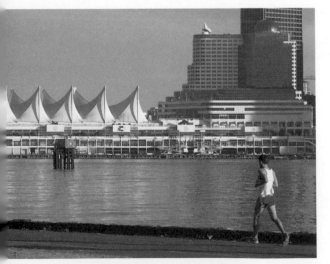

Road-running Essentials

Only the most basic running kit is required to get started as a road runner – shoes, socks, shorts and a top. Although all these items should be good quality and fully fit for purpose (*see* page 72), none of the more specialist wear required for trail running is needed.

City Breaks

Running in an urban environment can be every bit as exhilarating and enjoyable as a country run. There is always the opportunity to explore new corners of even the most familiar towns or cities, and if you take your running shoes on holiday, this can be an excellent way of familiarizing yourself with a new place. Local runners can be a great source of information.

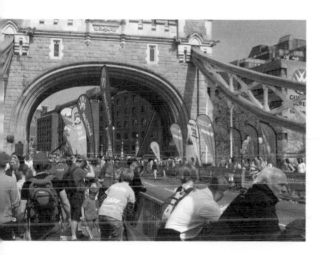

Follow the Crowd

Many of the world's greatest races take place on roads and in cities. Just think of the Great North Run (Newcastle to South Shields in the UK) or the London, New York and Berlin marathons. City races attract not only the greatest number of runners, but also the largest – and usually the loudest – crowds. Nothing is more motivating when participating in a race than a sea of waving spectators.

The Pros of City Running

- ✅ Unbroken, smooth running surfaces
- ✅ No sense of isolation for lone runners
- ✅ Help at hand if needed

The Cons of City Running

- ✅ Traffic and pollution
- ✅ Stopping to cross roads
- ✅ Crowds and rush hour

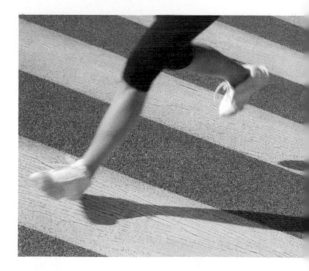

Trail Running

Trail running, or off-road running, refers to many things. Put simply, it encompasses anything that is not road running. Woods, hills, footpaths, bridleways and open pastures can all be explored with an incredible sense of freedom and adventure.

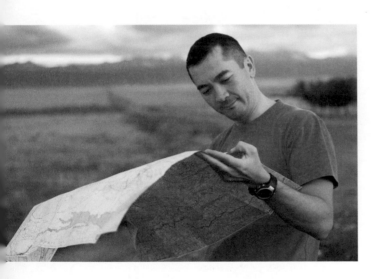

Find That Route

Online forums are a good place to start when looking for new places to explore off-road. Many runners post and share their own experiences, and these can be a useful source of information on where to go and, sometimes more importantly, where *not* to go. If you are looking to trail-blaze a new route, there is great pleasure to be had in studying large-scale maps and planning a run from scratch.

'Take Me Home!'

A GPS watch can be useful on new routes, as many feature a 'take me home' function that will allow you to retrace your steps if you become lost – but this is no substitute for good navigational skills; if in doubt, pack a map.

Top Tip

When exploring a new route, always tell someone roughly where you are intending to run to and how long you are likely to be.

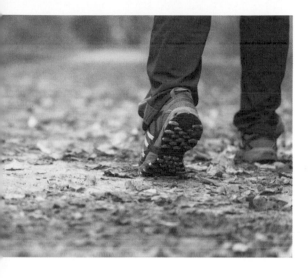

Kit Up

Some specialist kit for off-road running is recommended, and shoes designed for trail are essential (*see* page 56). Many runners head for the hills (and fields) more frequently during the winter months, as mud and a degree of adverse weather make for much of the fun. With this in mind, you are likely to require additional running clothing such as wind- and waterproof jacket, tights rather than shorts, plus base layers, hats and gloves. Do not let the weather spoil a good run.

The Pros of Trail Running

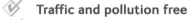

- Traffic and pollution free
- Sense of freedom
- More adventurous routes
- Greater mental challenge

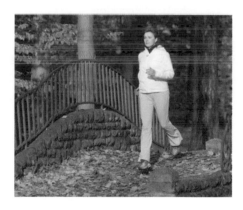

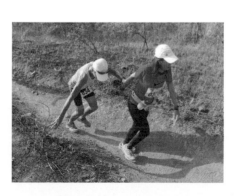

The Cons of Trail Running

- Uneven surfaces
- Isolation
- Navigation required
- Some additional kit required

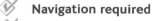
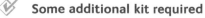

Training Runs

When it comes to training, there are many types of run to consider. Depending on your goals (which are likely to evolve with time), these could include everything from hills to speed work and increasingly long distances. Understanding your goals will help you determine what kinds of training runs you need to undertake.

Base Run

Every runner has a favourite local run, which could be anything from a 20-minute run around the block to a loop of 10 miles or more. This is likely to form the foundation of your base run – a regular, steady-paced and comfortable route that can be extended by an extra block or two if the mood takes you. It will generally be completed at a more-or-less constant pace.

Setting the Pace

If you run with a partner, a good rule of thumb is to keep your pace on a base run 'conversationally comfortable' – that is, you should be able to maintain a conversation without getting out of breath. If you are already a competitive runner and know your average pace for races, a base run should be completed at around 1.5 minutes per mile *slower* than this.

Interval Training

Interval training is the cornerstone for improving the speed at which you run. Although it can help you increase your pace on any run, it is particularly useful when training for distances under 10k.

Interval-training Techniques

There are many variations on this training technique, but, at its simplest, interval training involves running at a fast pace for a given length of time (or distance) followed by a longer interval of slower running. For example, after warming up, run at near-sprint speed for 30 seconds, slow to a gentle pace (sometimes called the 'recovery interval') and then repeat.

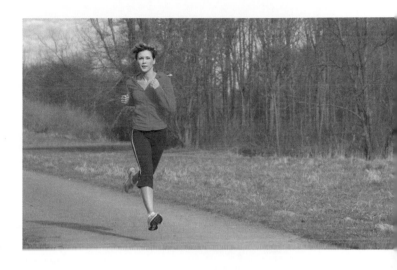

Benefits of Interval Training

Along with increased speeds, there are other benefits to interval training. Cardiovascular condition (heart/blood flow) will improve, along with many other factors that can otherwise adversely affect your running. The efficiency with which your body absorbs oxygen (known as VO2Max) – crucial to better running – may show rapid improvement with regular interval running.

Top Tip

Some runners find the repetition of interval training tedious; if you're one of these people, find someone to train with to add a competitive element to the sprints.

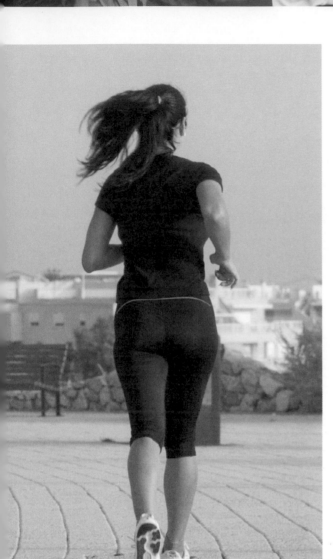

Fartlek Run

Fartlek, Swedish for 'speed play', is similar to interval training, but far less structured and rigorous. Instead of running for predetermined intervals of speed or distance, the fartlek technique involves bursts of higher speed, followed by slower recovery sections, more or less as the mood suits. Greater discipline can be introduced by running between regularly spaced markers such as lampposts.

Benefits of Fartlek Running

The fartlek technique may sound imprecise, but it shares many of the same benefits as interval training – increasing your running efficiency and ultimately your speed. Fartlek training is an excellent way of beginning this process; many new runners begin with more relaxed fartlek runs and then move on to more structured interval training as their technique and confidence grow.

Top Tip

Fartlek can be motivational, allowing you to challenge and reward yourself: 'If I can run hard to point X, I'll treat myself with a gentle run for five minutes ...' Go ahead – treat yourself.

Tempo Run

The tempo run, which varies in length from 20–50 minutes a week depending on your fitness and running schedule, is one of the most efficient ways of building both strength and speed. Tempo runs are simple runs of steady effort, and the key is to keep the pace *just* at the upper limit of your comfort zone. As your fitness and running improve, so too will the upper limits of that comfort zone.

Tempo running works by gradually pushing back the limits of your lactic threshold (LT), the point at which your muscles begin to feel fatigued. As with all training runs, it is vital to warm up slowly for 5–10 minutes before beginning a tempo run.

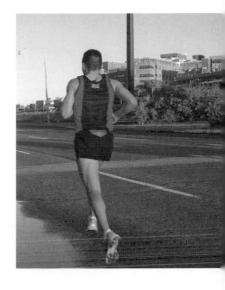

Hill Reps

The idea of hill reps is simple: run up a hill, run down, repeat ... But with a little variation, hill reps can be one of the most useful tools in a runner's box of tricks.

First and foremost, hill reps are an excellent way of training for an event that involves a lot of elevation. However, they also help with general running fitness and in building specific muscle groups. In particular, the downhill sections build strength through the quads (quadriceps), the upper leg muscles that serve as the body's natural shock absorbers. The quads are the most common area to suffer delayed onset muscle soreness (DOMS) a day or two after a hilly run, so mixing hill reps into your training – even once or twice a month – can help.

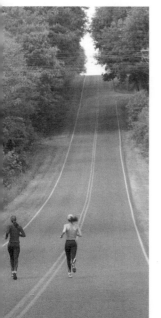

Top Tip

A heart rate monitor (HRM) is a good way of measuring progress with tempo, fartlek and interval running.

Sprint

Sprinting as part of general running – as opposed to the field event, which is a highly specialized area – is usually limited to two areas for most runners. It is used as part of a specific training exercise such as an interval run, or for a sprint finish at the end of a race.

Most runners, however inexperienced, can usually find the reserves for a sprint to the line at an organized event, regardless of the distance already covered. A cheering crowd and a rush of adrenaline can push even the most exhausted runner into a turn of speed that can surprise and delight.

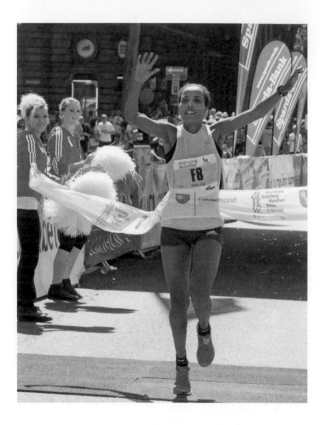

Be Aware

Two words of warning on the sprint finish. Firstly, as exhilarating as the final burst might feel, beware of injury. It is all too common for a runner to enjoy a well-paced and successful race only to injure themselves in the last 100 metres. Secondly, on general (non-race) runs, a sprint finish to your door might impress the neighbours, but a five-minute warm-down pace is better training. Sprinting and other speed work may not be suitable for the absolute beginner; as a general rule, endurance (how *far* you can run) will always come before how *fast*.

Long Run

A long run should be just that – long. However, this could mean 30 minutes or 30 miles, depending on your definition of 'long' and how your endurance increases as your training progresses. When planning a long run, bear two things in mind:

- ☑ **It should be longer than your base run (how much longer depends on your fitness and goals).**
- ☑ **It should be progressive, getting longer as the weeks pass.**

Increasing the Distance

Training for an event will probably involve increasing your long run gradually until it reaches the distance (or nearly so) of the race. As a general rule, you should increase the length of a run by no more than 10–15 per cent a week. Sudden large jumps in distance will greatly enhance the risk of injury and quickly set back your training.

Be Inspired

'Do a little more each day than you think you possibly can.'
Lowell Thomas, broadcaster and writer

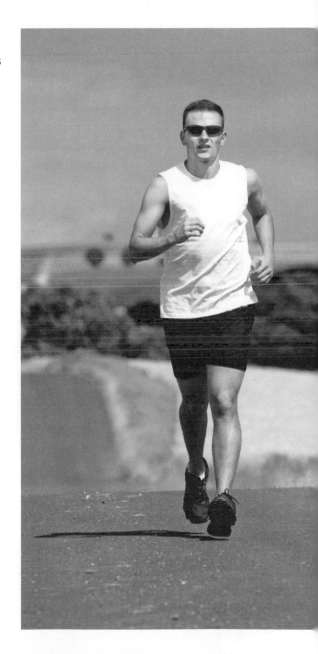

Recovery Run

Never underestimate the recuperative powers of a recovery run – a slow, gentle and (usually) short run in the days following either a particularly hard/long run or a race event. Recovery runs can still form part of a training programme; just because they are 'easy' miles, does not mean they do not count!

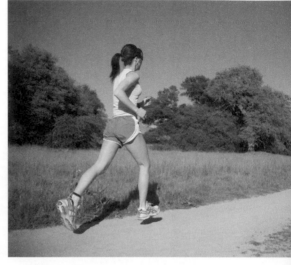

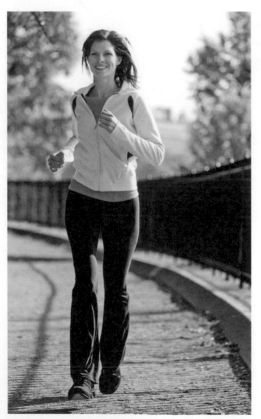

Benefits of the Recovery Run

Recovery runs work well in two ways:

- **Physical**: A slow, gentle run will shake out tight muscles and general stiffness, as well as helping to rid the body of toxins that may have accumulated during a long run.

- **Mental**: It is common to hear a first-time race competitor stagger into the arms of a loved one at the finish line and puff, 'I'll never run again!' The recovery run should both convince you that you *can* still run and remind you just how much you love it.

Checklist

- **Choose your distance**: Explore the many races, ranging from 5k to marathon (and beyond), listed online. With thousands to choose from, there is certain to be something to inspire.

- **Road or trail**: Although it does not have to be a clear-cut choice, most runners start out with a preference, so find out about them and decide which might work for you.

- **Choose your kit well**: Road and trail kit (especially shoes) are very different – make sure you have the right gear.

- **Is city running for you?** Consider the pros and cons carefully.

- **Safety**: Check that your route is safe and take all sensible precautions, especially when training at night.

- **Stay hydrated**: Check that you drink enough before and after training. Drink during training too, especially if it is a long or hot session.

- **Avoid injury**: Always warm up, cool down and stretch as part of your training routine.

Footwear

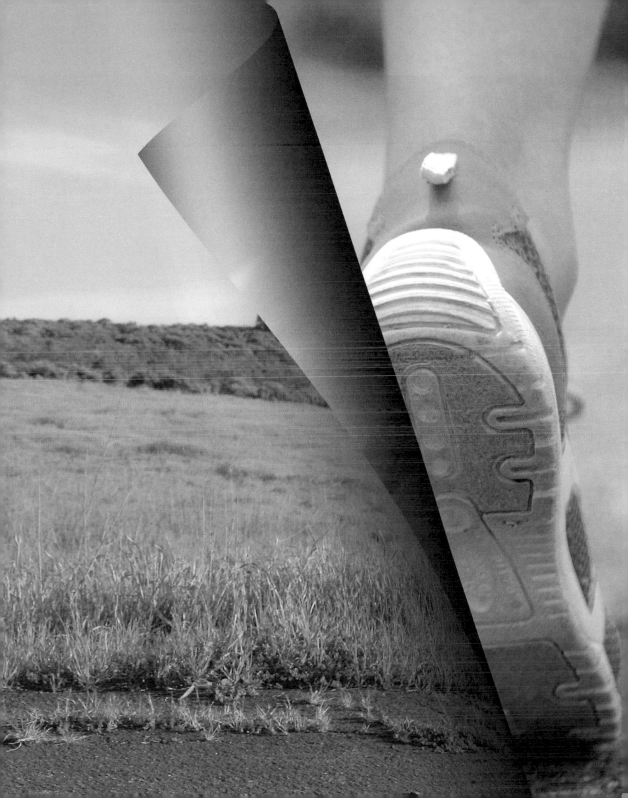

Getting It Right

The worst thing you can do as a new runner is choose the wrong pair of shoes; even the most experienced runners can occasionally be taken in by a combination of an attractive design and smart marketing. Spending a little time at the start of your running career learning some shoe (and foot) basics can save you a world of pain and poor performance later on.

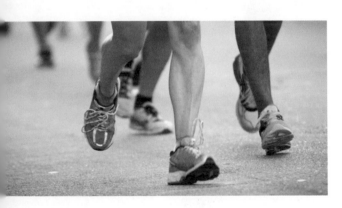

Hitting the Ground

The first question you should ask yourself is, 'What sort of feet do I have?' With the exception of so-called barefoot shoes (*see* page 57), most running shoes force a 'heel-strike' running action – one in which the heel hits the ground first, before rolling through the length of the foot and pushing back off through the toe.

Heel strike, Midfoot or Forefoot?

There are raging debates about whether heel strike is a natural style of running or merely one forced upon runners by the shoe industry. In time, you may find that you are a better midfoot or forefoot runner; there are advanced training techniques that aid this development, and switching to barefoot shoes can help.

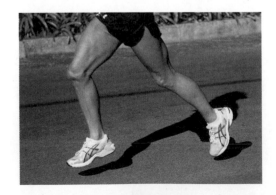

Pronation

Pronation Is the amount of sideways rolling motion your foot makes as it hits the ground, and every runner pronates to a degree. However, in overpronators the foot continues rolling inwards past the optimum point for efficient running, whilst in underpronators the foot does not roll enough. Both overpronation and underpronation can be corrected by the right shoes, and this is why it is important to buy them from a specialist running shop.

Understanding Your Arches

The arch of the foot (the upwards curve of the sole, part of the foot's mechanism for supporting the weight of the body) plays a role in pronation and thus the decision-making process for shoes. Runners with either high or particularly low arches (also called 'flat feet') will need shoes that compensate for this.

Getting Support

A good running shop will talk new runners through the complexities of shoe types, so you don't need to worry too much about fully understanding terms such as 'high arches' or 'pronation'. However, it can be useful to familiarize yourself with the four main options for correcting these running characteristics.

Top Tip

Uncorrected pronation not only makes running less efficient but can also lead to many of the most common running injuries.

Neutral Cushioning

These are intended for runners with higher arches and with little pronation. They are designed to offer greater midsole support or cushioning, which compensates for the lack of 'foot roll'. They can also be useful for midfoot and forefoot runners.

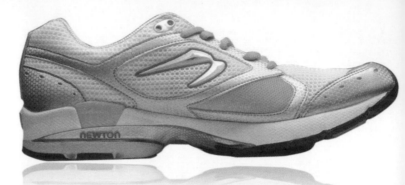

Newton's 'Sir Isaac' running shoe is a neutral-cushioning shoe designed for runners seeking to ease transition from heel striking to midfoot running.

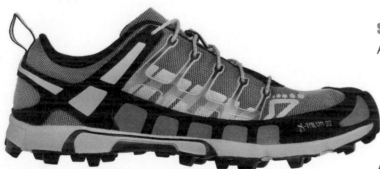

Inov-8's 'X-Talon™ 212' off-road shoe is designed to offer 'the optimum combination of minimal weight, stability and grip'.

Stability

Average pronators with normal or slightly low arches should look for stability running shoes. They offer varying degrees of cushioning, support and stability, so finding the pair that best suits your style of running is key.

Performance

Designed for the lucky few who are considered 'biomechanically efficient' (having a natural ability to run in terms of foot strike and roll), performance shoes offer some degree of both cushioning and support, but they are generally lighter than 'normal' running shoes.

Motion Control

Runners with very low arches and average to severe overpronation are best suited to motion-control shoes, which are more extreme versions of stability shoes.

Anatomy of a Shoe

Modern running shoes are precision-built from a large number of individual components, each designed to perform a specific function and to work in harmony with each other. Manufacturers' websites should detail all the technical aspects of their shoes.

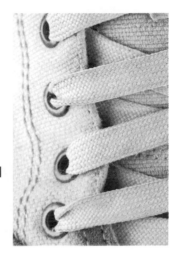

Jargon-buster

Here are some of the main terms you will find when researching running shoes.

- ✅ **Eyelets**: The holes that the laces run through.

- ✅ **Heel**: The first point of contact for many runners. The heel is often rounded to aid forward motion and may be made of a variety of materials, from gel to air pockets.

- ✅ **Collar:** The soft inside top rear of the shoe that supports the ankle and provides protection for the Achilles tendon.

- ✅ **Heel counter:** A rigid, moulded support inside the shoe that cradles the heel.

- ✅ **Heel tab**: This extends upwards from the heel counter at the rear of the shoe to hold the heel firmly in place. It often has a cutout area called an 'Achilles notch' to reduce direct pressure on the Achilles tendon.

- ✅ **Midsole**: This provides primary protection from the impact force of each foot strike. Although the midsole is usually made of foam, some manufacturers use special gels or air pockets.

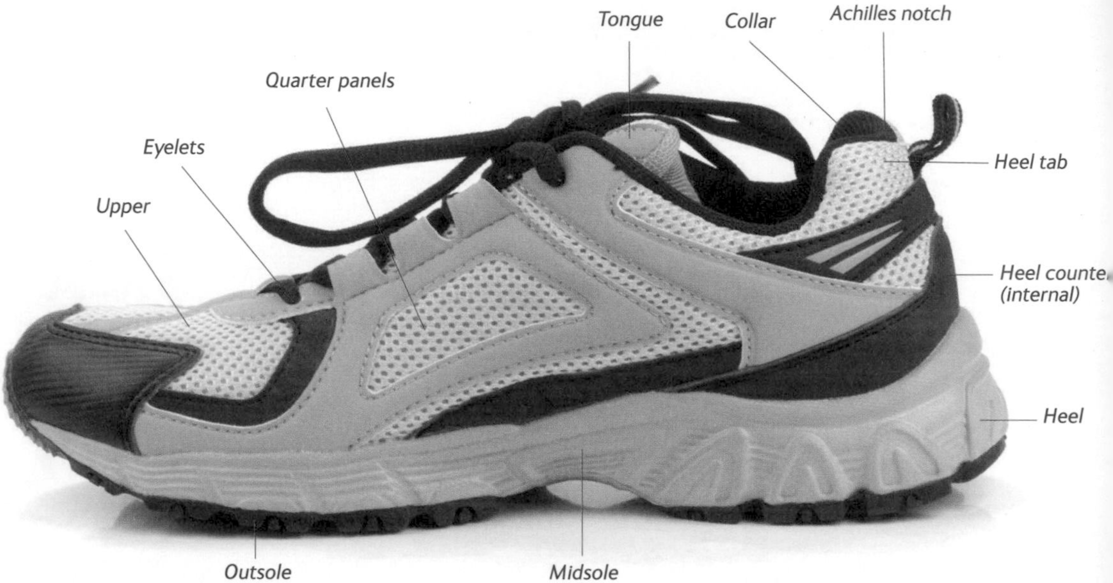

Tongue
Collar
Achilles notch
Quarter panels
Eyelets
Heel tab
Upper
Heel counter (internal)
Heel
Outsole
Midsole

☑ **Outsole**: The outsole is the bit that hits the ground (normally *after* the heel); it both provides structure to the shoe and gives traction on the running surface.

☑ **Quarter panels**: These are the sides of the shoe. They may include a small piece of mesh to reduce weight and add ventilation.

☑ **Footbed**: A removable insert that helps the shoe to fit snugly. It can usually be removed to aid drying.

☑ **Tongue**: The tongue sits between the laces and the upper foot. It may be 'gusted' (connected at the sides) to reduce the amount of water that can get in.

☑ **Upper**: This is the top part of the shoe that encases the foot. Like the quarter panels, these may incorporate a degree of mesh venting.

The Three Main Types

Besides specialist track shoes (with spikes), there are only three main types of shoe from which to choose: road, trail and the relatively new phenomenon of barefoot shoes. Each is designed for a specific purpose, so bear this in mind when making your decision. Seek impartial advice on the pros and cons of manufacturers and the latest designs by looking in running magazines and online forums.

Road Shoes

Road shoes are especially designed for running on hard surfaces. Some may be suitable for a small amount of trail or off-road running, but the quickest way to destroy your shoes is by using them for anything other than their intended purpose. The road shoes you choose will depend on a wide range of variables, the most important of which is your natural running style. This should be checked and advised upon by a specialist retailer.

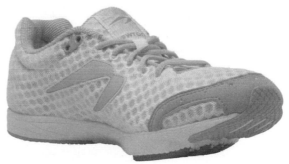

Newton's 'MV²' road shoe is designed to provide protection for running on hard surfaces.

Avoid Fashion

The price of road shoes varies enormously, but expect to pay anything from £40/$60 to in excess of £100/$160. To some degree, you get what you pay for, but do not be fooled into simply thinking that the more you pay, the better the shoe. There is more than a dash of fashion in running, and you will always pay a premium for the big-name shoes and the latest designs. Many of these will be packed with a multitude of technical-sounding extras that often serve little purpose for the majority of day-to-day running.

Trail Shoes

Trail shoes not only have to fulfil your basic needs in terms of cushioning and stability, they also have to perform a number of additional tasks, including protecting the toe and sole from uneven surfaces and delivering enhanced traction for wet and muddy conditions.

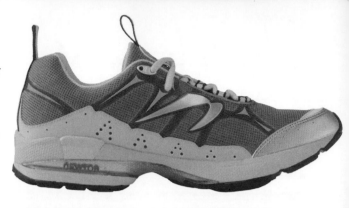

Newton's 'Momentum' is a trail shoe designed for all types of terrain.

Getting a Grip

Trail running inevitably means uneven and often wet terrains; your shoes need to be up to the job of keeping you upright and providing enough traction to move you forward. Different manufacturers use a range of tread styles to achieve this, ranging from quite flat car tyre-style treads to large studs (or 'lugs') or even additional metal spikes. Low-profile treads provide good all-round traction, but they are unlikely to stand up to the very worst conditions. Conversely, shoes with really large lugs (resembling football boots) will handle more gruelling terrain but can skid on firmer or more compact surfaces.

Multitasking

Trail shoes with low-profile lugs will allow *some* degree of road running to get you to the start of your off-road route. If you are likely to be running multi-terrain – a mix of trail, path and road – then choose a pair without large lugs.

Top Tip

If the price looks too good to be true, perhaps it is. The internet is a haven for bogus products and counterfeit running shoes. Beware!

Barefoot Shoes

Nothing sounds more contradictory than a barefoot shoe, but over the last few years this running revolution has been transformed from a niche market – initially written off by many as a fad – to a massive industry with growing scientific backing. One of the sparks that ignited this quantum leap in shoe design was Christopher McDougall's book *Born to Run*, a highly recommended read even for the most novice runner.

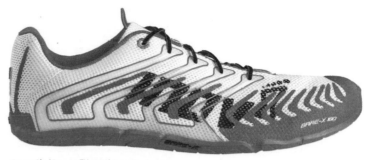

Inov-8's 'Bare-X™ 180' barefoot shoe

Natural Style

Barefoot shoes are little more than gloves for the feet, providing minimum padding against underfoot forces and, crucially, having no built-up heel, to encourage a more mid- to forefoot running style. This, proponents claim, is a more 'biomechanically efficient' way of running, far more in line with the way we were intended to run in an evolutionary sense. Research certainly seems to support this claim, and barefoot runners are undeniably evangelical about the advantages.

Top Tip

Trail versions of barefoot shoes are now available, featuring a greater degree of traction and protection. These are an excellent option for tentative runners to test the barefoot water.

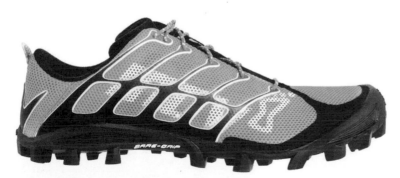

Inov-8's 'Bare-Grip™ 200' barefoot trail shoe

Buying and Caring For Your Shoes

Everyone knows that the internet is awash with bargains, but when it comes to shopping for running shoes there can be no substitute for the expert help and advice – combined with the opportunity to test-drive the shoes – that can be found in a specialist running shop. Equally important is knowing how to take care of them once you have made your choice.

The Key to Shoe Shopping

Below are some top tips for successful shoe shopping.

- **Seek out the experts**: Always shop at a specialist running shop.

- **Take advice**: Have staff carefully check your running style.

- **Buy in the afternoon**: Test shoes later in the day, when your feet are likely to have swollen *slightly*.

- **Avoid the heat**: Your feet may be *too* swollen on excessively hot days.

- **Test the shoes**: Use the shop's treadmill to try out the shoes you like before making your final selection.

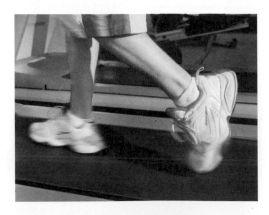

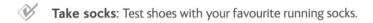

- **Take socks:** Test shoes with your favourite running socks.

- **Take your time:** Spend time making a choice, and *never* feel obliged to buy.

- **Look for instant comfort:** Shoes should feel comfortable straight out of the box.

Be Inspired

'Don't take anyone else's definition of success as your own.'
Jacqueline Briskin, author

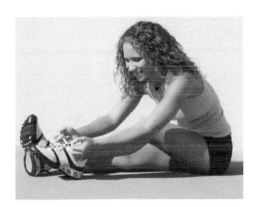

Love Your Shoes

Most people claim that good running shoes will last in the region of 500 miles. Of course, there are many factors that will add to the general wear and tear of even the toughest of shoes (not least your running style), so it's important to know how to look after your shoes, to extend their life span. It is also important to understand when to say goodbye to a much-loved pair.

The Good Care Guide

Taking a few simple steps to look after your shoes can extend their life span.

- **Do not delay:** As soon as possible after a run, sponge clean with warm water and only *very* mild detergent.

- **Dry naturally:** Air dry (or stuff with scrunched newspaper); never be tempted to dry on a radiator or in front of a fire.

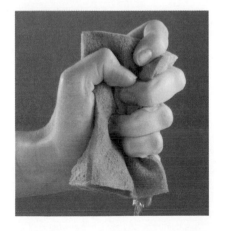

- ☑ **Remove insoles**: Take out the insoles or footbeds and leave to air dry.

- ☑ **Keep clean**: Remove dried mud with a soft, dry brush.

- ☑ **Keep safe**: Store in a cupboard away from direct sunlight and extremes of heat.

- ☑ **Do not multitask**: Keep running shoes for running, not the gym and not for gardening!

Signs of Retirement

Look out for the first stages of wear and tear to give yourself plenty of time to choose and buy replacements. Purchasing a new pair of shoes when there are still a few miles left in the old ones means you can alternate pairs to get used to your latest purchase.

- ☑ **Eyes**: Make a quick, regular visual check. External wear is often a sign of internal problems. Place shoes on a tabletop and look carefully at the wear around the heel and the outer midsole; wrinkles and creases can be a sign of compressed cushioning.

- ☑ **Fingers**: Pinch and press around the toe to test how much protection remains; it should spring back into shape without creases. Remove the insole and press one finger on to the midsole beneath; if it does not spring back, the cushioning is going.

- ☑ **Legs**: If ankles, legs and knees are feeling more fatigued than usual, or you have begun to suffer mild injuries (such as the early signs of shin splints), it is more than likely that your shoes are destined for the bin.

Top Tip

Many sports and running shops have recycling bins for retired shoes – a great way of supporting charities and avoiding landfill.

Checklist

☑ **Trail or road:** Shoes are designed for specific terrains; choose your shoes to fit your routes.

☑ **Check pronation:** Always have a specialist running shop identify your running style.

☑ **Know your type:** Neutral-cushioning, stability, motion-control and performance shoes need to suit your foot's natural design.

☑ **Beware bargains:** Counterfeit shoes are more common than you might think. Always buy from a reputable outlet.

☑ **Multi-terrain running:** Look for trail shoes with low-profile lugs to mix trail and *some* road running.

☑ **Experiment:** Barefoot running is increasingly popular and can improve your running style. It adds variety to your routine too.

☑ **Buying shoes:** Shop in the afternoon; take your time and test *thoroughly*.

☑ **Replace worn shoes:** Nothing causes more injuries than old, badly worn shoes. Check regularly for signs of wear and tear.

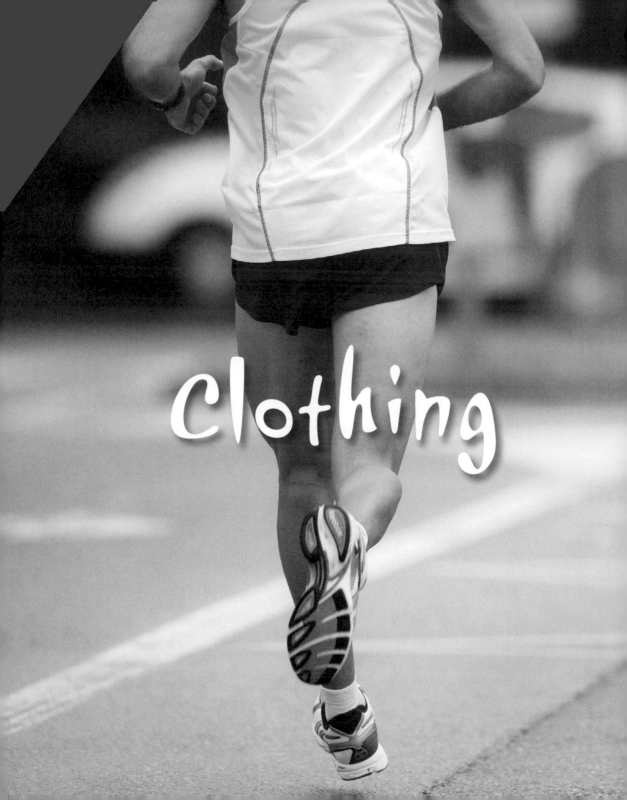

Clothing

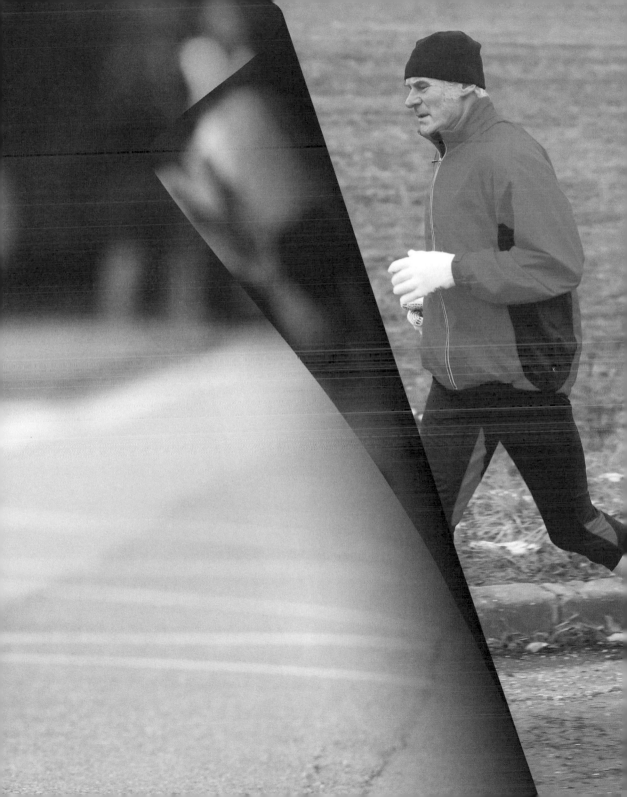

Choosing Running Clothes

At its simplest, running requires little more than shoes, socks, shorts and a top – either long-sleeved or T-shirt. However, in the same way that it is important to spend time and care in selecting the right running shoes, picking the correct clothing to go with them will pay dividends in the long run. This section gives you some starting points for choosing the right running clothes.

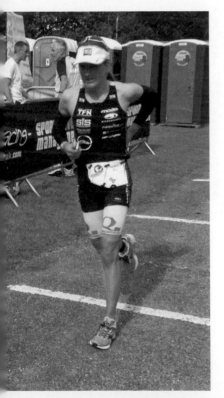

Count the Cost

At first glance, it might appear that 'technical' running clothes, those made from the latest and greatest modern materials, and with specialist designs, are too expensive. This applies to almost all sports clothes – everything from the socks upwards. Certainly, this type of clothing is considerably more expensive than the basic shorts and tops available from high-street shops or discount stores.

However, bear in mind the long-term outlay you're likely to make on your running clothes. Cheap apparel will usually wear out far more quickly than the costlier gear. A cheap T-shirt will be unwearable within a few months, whereas a quality running top will last you many years.

Material Factors

In addition to its short life span, cheaper clothing is inadvisable because of the material used. This type of clothing is unlikely to either wick away moisture and/or feature breathable materials, which can make the running experience uncomfortable at best – and pretty much unbearable at worst.

Wicking

Wicking is the ability of a fabric to draw moisture (sweat) away from the skin. Unlike cotton – which can absorb more than seven per cent of its weight in water – modern sports fabrics employ a range of techniques, most notably one called 'capillary pressure', to keep the skin dry.

Breathability

Working hand-in-hand with wicking, breathability is a material's capacity to help regulate body temperature. Simply think of it as a one-way system that allows sweaty moisture out but does not allow cold air in.

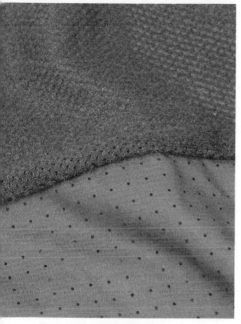

Breathable jacket material

Key Advice

- ✔ **Never wear cotton.**
- ✔ **Check for wicking and breathability.**
- ✔ **Choose light colours for sunny days.**
- ✔ **Look for UV protection.**
- ✔ **Select high-visibility and reflective panels for safety.**
- ✔ **Buy cheap – buy twice.**

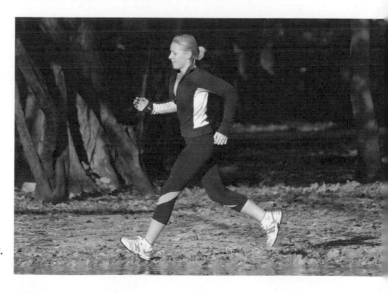

Summer Basics

Running on a bright summer's day can bring an unrivalled sense of wellbeing, but if your running clothes are not up to the job, that sense of joy will be short-lived. Most runners buy their clothing with dry, sunny conditions in mind – only later becoming more adventurous with midwinter runs – so most clothing is suitable for summer weather.

T-shirts and Shorts

T-shirts and tops designed for summer running tend to be brighter and more colourful, but it is crucial to balance the head and the heart when choosing the right kit. Always check that the material used in the T-shirt or top offers the best possible wicking and breathability. Remember too that a slightly looser fit (not baggy) will help you keep cool.

Buy slightly looser-fitting shorts for summer running, too. These will help air circulate and prevent sweating and chafing. However, do not be tempted by very short shorts – the more leg on show, the greater the risk of sunburn.

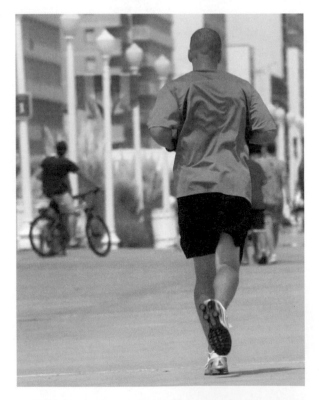

Sun Shields

Both shorts and tops should
incorporate some sun shield within
the material, so look for fabrics that
offer both UVA and UVB protection.
These are the long- and short-wave
rays that lead to sunburn and the
risk of skin cancers.

Beware the Sun!

Summer running should be all about
keeping it simple, so don't load yourself
up with all manner of extra kit and
sportswear. Shorts, shoes, socks and a
T-shirt are plenty – but running in high
temperatures on sunny days without
a hat can be disastrous.

Hat Style

Personal preference will play a big
part in your hat selection, but always
remember that a hat should serve two
purposes on summer runs: protecting

Be Inspired

'All it takes is all you got!'
Marc Davis, track runner

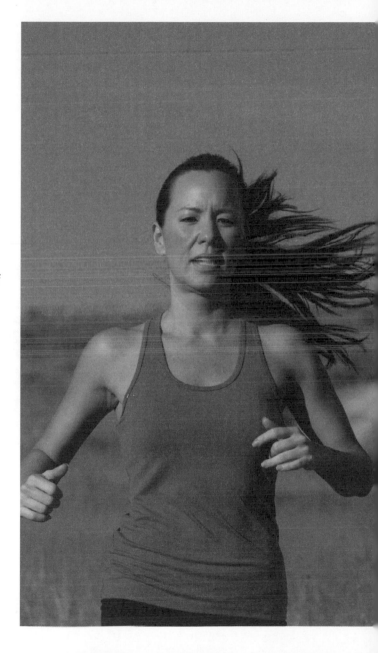

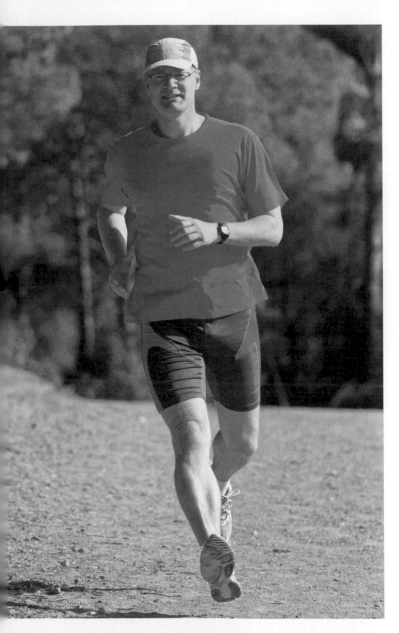

your head from the sun and keeping the sun out of your eyes. Poker-player style visors will block out the glare, but will do nothing to protect the top of your head. Instead, look for baseball-style caps, preferably with UVA/UVB protection material. Check the length of the peak – too short and it will be pointless, too long and it may bounce annoyingly with every stride. Mesh venting on the sides will help you keep a cool head.

Cooling Your Feet

Your feet are far more likely to sweat and swell up during a hot, summer run, and this increases the chances of developing blisters. Every care should be taken to keep your feet as cool and comfortable as possible. Running socks designed especially for summer training are usually shorter and have less padding, as well as having the best wicking to ensure that sweat is kept away from the skin.

Winter Basics

Many new runners are reluctant to head out when the seasons change for the worse, but running on a cold, bright winter's day has its own charms. Even running in rain and snow can be hugely invigorating and, as long as your clothes are fit for the weather, you will quickly discover the joy of year-round training. Besides being comfortable, winter running gear should serve two purposes: it should keep you at just the right temperature and keep the weather on the outside.

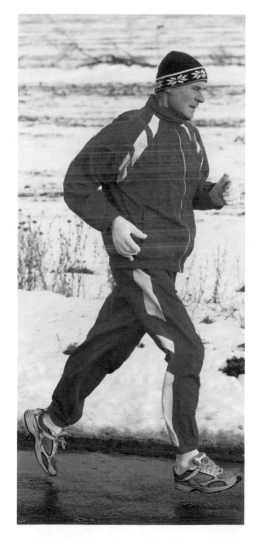

Temperature Control

One of the most common mistakes – even amongst experienced runners – is overestimating how cold a run will be. Put on multiple layers of clothing, hats, gloves and even scarves, and you'll regret the decision within a mile or two. Modern sports materials are designed to regulate your temperature; this includes the ability to trap warm air between the skin and the clothing, which acts as an inbuilt thermal layer.

Base Layers

In extremely cold conditions, particularly when there is a biting wind, consider wearing a base layer beneath your running top. However, you should make sure that each layer has good breathability and that the layer closest to the skin can still effectively wick away sweat.

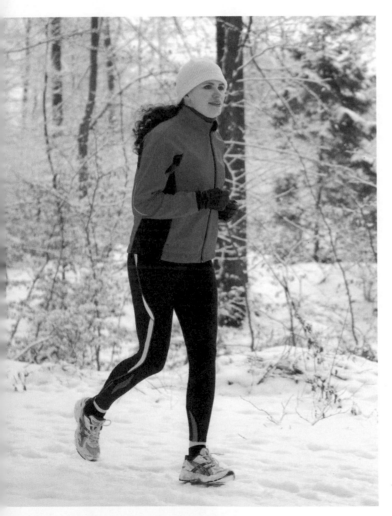

Top Layers

If a base layer feels too warm, try a light running jacket over your top instead. Many of these are designed to reduce the impact of cold winds and have the added advantage that they can be unzipped for ventilation as required. A degree of waterproofing in jackets is also typical, but do not expect the kind of full protection a much heavier hiking jacket would provide. Getting wet (often through to the skin) is all part of winter running, but as long as your tops, shorts and socks have comfortable seams, this should not be a problem.

Top Tip

When you start a winter's run, you should just be able to feel the cold. Feeling warm as soon as you set out is a sure sign of overheating ahead.

Wet Winter Feet

Some running socks incorporate a fully waterproof layer or membrane. These work exceptionally well if you run in shoes with plenty of mesh (generally lighter-weight shoes), but be aware that if water does get inside – for example, over the top in deep puddles – it will be trapped inside and may cause blisters. It is usually better to just choose slightly thicker, well-wicking socks and avoid puddles as far as possible! Socks made from a mix of merino wool and silk are particularly luxurious; consider buying a spare pair to pamper your feet.

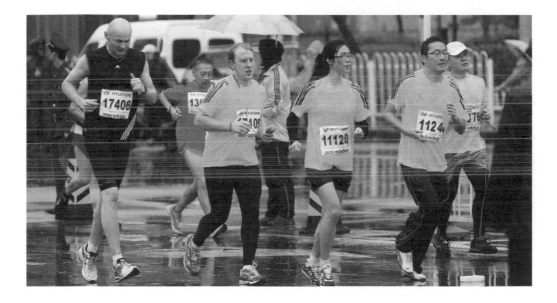

Gaiters

Waterproof gaiters, similar to trail gaiters (see page 74) but made from water-repellent materials, can be useful on wet runs to stop water trickling down the legs and into the tops of shoes or soaking the tops of your socks.

Top Tip

Some winter running jackets have additional vents that can be unzipped either at the sides or under the arms to tailor the amount of heat they retain.

Trail Clothing

Leaving the roads and pavements behind for the joys of off-road and trail running can be a truly liberating experience and a great way of exploring new areas. As with your running shoes, though, it is important to ensure that your general running kit is up to the job.

Fit for Purpose

Much of your regular running wear will be able to cope with a certain amount of light off-road action, but if you find that trail is your thing (and it can be really addictive once you've tried it), then you'll probably want – and need – a number of specialist items that will make your trail running more enjoyable, comfortable and safer.

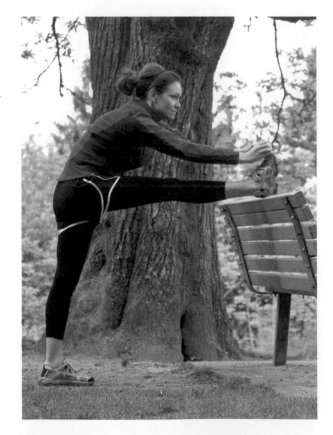

Be Inspired

'We may train or peak for a certain race, but running is a lifetime sport.'
Alberto Salazar, marathon runner

Long is Better

When trail running, your legs will be best
protected by longer shorts or tights –
depending on the terrain you are running
through. It is more than likely that you will
encounter any combination of vegetation,
nettles and low-settled twigs and branches, which
(especially if you are behind another runner) have
a tendency to lash back painfully against the legs.
Cover your legs well, but avoid baggy clothing
that might snag on branches. Similarly, longer or
full-length sleeves on your running top will
protect your arms.

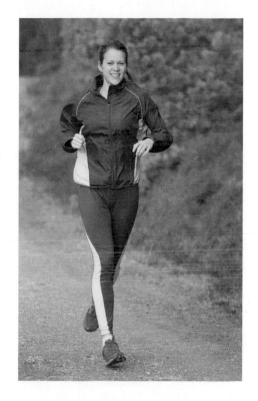

Foot Protection

Trail-specific socks are widely available, and there
are two main options:

✓ **Long socks:** These can be almost knee-length, and are useful if you are wearing shorts
and want to add further protection to the lower legs.

✓ **Ankle socks:** If you are wearing running tights, choose a shorter or anklet sock that has
been designed for off-road running.

Sock Style

Depending on your needs and running style, trail socks may incorporate more padding than
your normal road sock, because trail is invariably more uneven and undulating, and likely to
punish your feet more. Look for socks with the greatest amount of wicking; off-road, they will
not just be dealing with sweat but probably mud and puddles too.

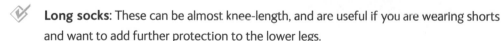

Trail Gaiters

Specialist gaiters, most of which slip over the shoe and lower leg/ankle and are secured below the heel, can be invaluable for keeping out tiny stones and other hazards that would otherwise lead to rubbing and blisters. Some manufacturers produce socks that incorporate a gaiter element as an all-in-one solution, and these are excellent for beach and sand running as well as trail running.

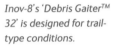

Inov-8's 'Debris Gaiter™ 32' is designed for trail-type conditions.

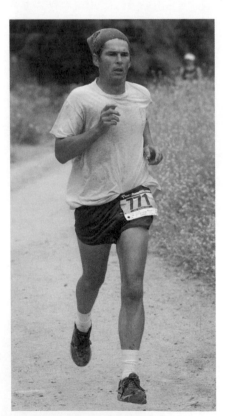

Trail Extras

If you're planning on running in the gloom of the woods, consider buying a runner's head-torch. Check these for comfort before you buy, making sure the lamp element is not so heavy that it will bounce uncontrollably, and remember that the torch will be heavier once it has batteries in it (these are unlikely to be fitted in the display model in the shop).

A bandana can be useful for trail running. For normal use, it will keep sweat out of your eyes and even offer some degree of protection from backlashing or low-hanging twigs. Better still, it doubles as a cleaning cloth for wiping trail grime from sports watches, MP3 players and mud-splattered faces.

Your Running Wardrobe

Your running requirements are likely to change over time, as your running progresses. As such, you may find that, in addition to the basics, you are drawn to a host of additional running wear. Base layers, running jackets, hats and gloves can open up year-round runs and introduce you to the joys of running in even the worst weather. Compression wear may help you both train harder and recover faster.

T-shirts

Along with shoes, socks and shorts, a good T-shirt is one of the most basic items on the runner's checklist. Your T-shirts can say a lot about you; as your running progresses and you take your first tentative steps at organized events, you will be amazed how quickly your collection of free T-shirts grows. However, there are important choices to make when it comes to buying your first running shirt.

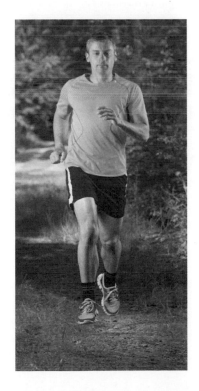

Avoid Cotton

When choosing a T-shirt, consider the material and, as with other clothing, never be tempted to run in cotton (many event T-shirts are cotton, so save them for the beach). Cotton soaks up sweat or rain and, when it does, it becomes heavy, causing it to rub and chafe. Men's nipples are particularly prone to chafing, as they don't have the added protection of a bra. Soaked cotton is also particularly bad at helping to maintain your body temperature.

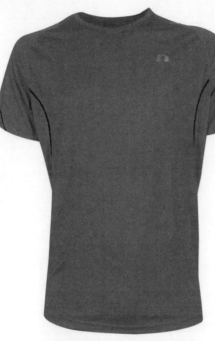

Newline's 'Coolmax' T-shirt uses special microfibre yarns designed to provide good wicking and evaporation.

Good Fabrics

Sportswear manufacturers all have their own patented materials, including Coolmax and Dri-Fit. These all do more or less the same thing: they wick water away from the skin through a one-way layer to the T-shirt's surface, where it harmlessly evaporates. These materials – and therefore the T-shirts – are generally more expensive than cotton alternatives, but are absolutely worth the investment for the comfort they bring to a run.

Added Value

Beyond the golden rule of never running in cotton, your choices are endless, and the extra features incorporated by different manufacturers become much more a matter of personal preference. However, there are a few additions that really do add value.

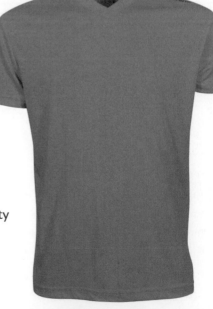

UV protection will defend against the sun's harmful rays, whilst the most advanced (and expensive) fabrics can regulate your temperature by reacting to changes in heat.

Reflective patches and bright colours will help with visibility and there are even T-shirts available with inbuilt channels through which you can run your headphone cables!

If you are particularly prone to sweating, then look for materials that have an inbuilt antibacterial element. This will help reduce smell and can extend the life of your T-shirt considerably.

Shorts

Available in a variety of styles and materials, most shorts will be designed either for men or women. Some unisex makes are available, but, as they have been created to fit neither gender specifically, they are best avoided.

The Long and the Short of It

Length of shorts is really down to personal preference, but, as a general rule, longer shorts give greater protection from twigs and other trail hazards for off-road runs, as well as offering better coverage on sunny days. Truly short shorts are generally the preserve of short-distance speed runners, so choosing something that feels good and allows plenty of room is a more important consideration.

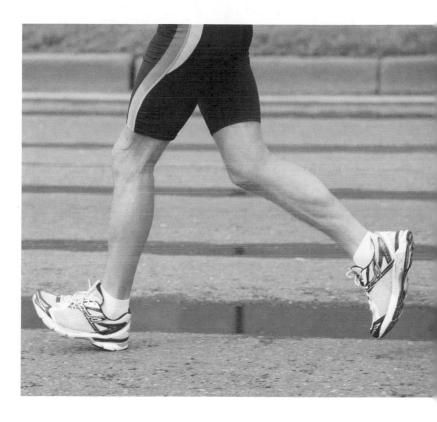

Top Tip

Light colours reflect the sun and keep you cooler; black tops may add a dash of 'ninja cool', but actually make you hotter.

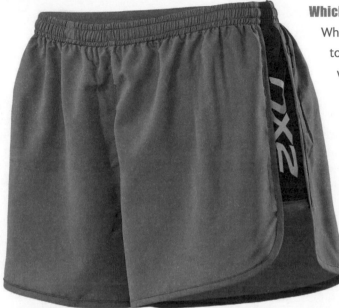

2XU's run shorts use their light 'VAPOR' fabric, designed to have efficient wicking properties and freedom of movement.

Which Material?

When choosing your shorts – as with tops – it is best to avoid cotton, which performs badly when it comes to regulating heat and tends to absorb moisture, leading to rubbing and discomfort. Nylon-based shorts also under-perform and will cling uncomfortably to sweaty legs and bottoms. Most major sportswear manufacturers have bespoke combinations of materials (many with bewildering semi-scientific names), but, as long as you remember to avoid cotton and cheap nylon, most materials will serve you well.

Be Inspired

'Don't bother just to be better than your contemporaries or predecessors. Try to be better than yourself.'
William Faulkner, author

Gender Specifics

Most men's shorts incorporate an integrated liner, which should be soft, wick away moisture and sweat efficiently, and provide sufficient support so that separate underwear is unnecessary. The idea of 'running commando' (without underwear) can strike fear into the heart of a new runner, but give it a go – normal underwear beneath shorts is far more likely to chafe in areas that you really will not appreciate. Not to mention the feeling of freedom that comes with running in shorts alone!

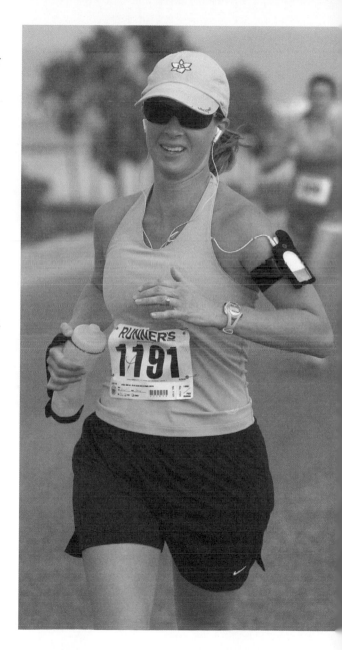

On the other hand, women's shorts rarely feature liners, so choosing the right underwear is essential. Sports knickers are available – something akin to those old school-day ones but most women find that simply wearing a comfortable, *larger* pair of knickers on a run is all that is required. Avoid anything too skimpy (thongs are not the right underwear for running) and, as with the material for shorts, avoid cotton and nylon knickers.

Extra Features

One or two additional features are worth considering when it comes to shorts. If you intend to run at night or on darker winter days, look for reflective detailing in your shorts, to make you more visible. A tiny patch of reflective material won't do much good (although it's better than nothing), so look for a substantial reflective down the sides of the shorts, along with some detailing on the bottom.

Many shorts also incorporate a small pocket. This can be useful for keeping your front door key safe, but avoid overloading even the most generously proportioned pocket – heavy shorts make for a heavy run. If you intend to carry extras with you, such as gels or bars, buy a pack or bum bag instead.

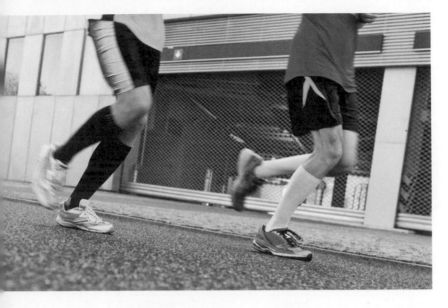

Socks

There is certainly far more to running socks than you might think at first, and no matter how good your shoes are, they would be nothing without the right choice of sock to slip in them. You will find socks on the market for every running occasion, terrain, season and style. So which should you choose?

Avoid Cotton – Again!

Cheap cotton socks should be rejected outright. Cotton will draw up sweat, quickly become uncomfortable and inevitably result in blisters. Most manufacturers have specially designed materials, but the most important features of a material are the ability to wick moisture and breathability.

Besides synthetic wicking materials, there are also several natural fabrics that perform the same function. Merino wool (from the sheep of the same name, prized for its luxuriously soft fleece) offers natural wicking and heat-control properties. Look for socks made from this mixed with a percentage of silk for a truly pampering experience, but be aware that they can be hot on summer runs.

Newline's 'Seamless Socklets' aim to reduce the risk of toe pain or blisters due to seams.

Padding It Out

When choosing socks, also consider the type of terrain you'll be running on. Trail running, particularly routes with lots of inclines, will be more punishing on the feet, so additional protection can be an advantage.

The degree of padding on socks varies from virtually zero to designs that look more like a hybrid slipper. If you are prone to blisters, try a pair with greater padding around the toes; if you find your soles ache during and after a run, look for socks with some degree of padding along the length.

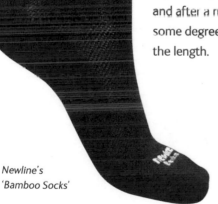

Newline's 'Bamboo Socks'

Newline's '2 Layer' socks have an inner and outer sock and toe protection seam.

Top Tip

Consider bamboo socks. Fabric made from bamboo is environmentally friendly, naturally wicks, controls temperature and even possesses natural antibacterial properties. Help your feet and the planet!

Left and Right

Some types of sock are 'anatomically correct' — that is, they are designed specifically for either the left foot or the right foot (they will probably be marked 'L' and 'R'). Again, these technical socks are generally more expensive, but, as our left and right feet are rough mirror images of each other, rather than identical, this approach does make sense.

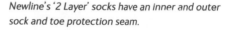

Tights

Female runners are unlikely to have an issue with donning a pair of tights, but men might be more reluctant to consider this piece of running apparel, even with the knowledge that tights can add a super-hero look to their running! However, in the winter months particularly, running tights can add considerable warmth to your outfit, and even in the summer tights can be preferable for trail running, when nettles and low-level twigs can inflict a nasty sting on bare legs.

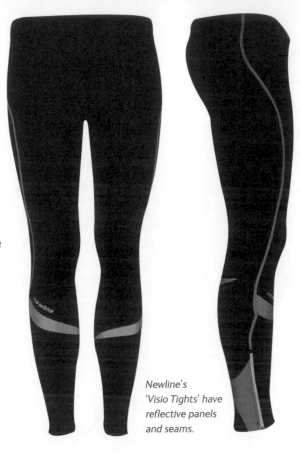

Newline's 'Visio Tights' have reflective panels and seams.

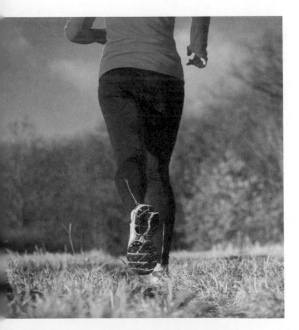

Fantastic Elastic

Running tights are generally made from a combination of synthetic materials, including a percentage of stretchy spandex or elastine, which give the garments both their figure-hugging form and the right amount of manoeuvrability. As with any running material that is going to sit directly against the skin, always look for tights that offer wicking properties to draw sweat away from the body.

Stirrups

Some tights incorporate stirrups that slip inside the shoes and under the foot to stop the bottom of the tight legs from riding up. Although whether or not you choose tights with stirrups is entirely personal choice, be aware that stirrups will have an impact on the fit and comfort of both your shoes and socks, and can lead to rubbing around the ankles. Because of their elastic qualities, tights are unlikely to move up to any great degree even without stirrups.

When it comes to comfort, also check carefully how flat the seams on tights feel, particularly around the groin. Even the best wicking tights will chafe if the seams are too bulky or appear misplaced for your physique.

Additional Features

Small pockets are often incorporated into running tights – usually at the back on the waistband. These are useful for holding keys, but, as with shorts, do not be tempted to overload them beyond this point.

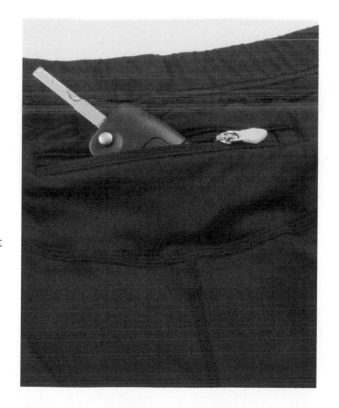

Tights that include UV protection are becoming much more commonplace, and these can protect against the sun's rays. Unfortunately it is rare to find running tights in anything other than dark colours (usually black), so the general advice about selecting lighter colours to keep you cool on summer runs does not apply here.

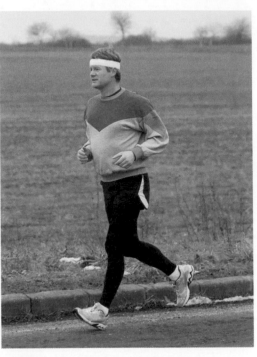

Top Tip

Feel self-conscious about tights? Many people like to wear loose-fitting shorts over the top of their tights to protect their modesty!

Bras

Choosing the right running bra is critical – the wrong type of bra will not only make your run an uncomfortable one, but can lead to longer-term shoulder and back problems. Unsupported or poorly supported breasts will also put strain on the Cooper's ligament, the connective tissues that help maintain shape and structure.

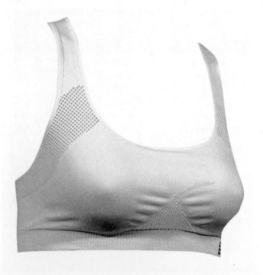

There are two types of running bra:

 Compression bras: These slip on over the head without clips and hold the breasts flat to the chest. However, they are really only recommended for the smaller form (nothing over a B cup).

 Encapsulation bras: These look similar to regular bras, in that they hold each breast separately, and they are best suited to supporting larger breasts.

Trying before buying is essential with running bras, and having one professionally fitted can make all the difference. Start out by trying on a running bra in your regular size and then stepping up or down from there. Make sure that the fit is snug – you should not be able to fit more than one finger inside the strap or cup – but not too tight or restrictive.

Base Layers

For midwinter runs, base layers fit below regular shorts and tops to add warmth. With varying degrees of thermal properties, base layers can be made from a range of materials and, in addition to the heat that they generate, a further benefit comes from the layer of air that is trapped between them and the outer layer.

Seams

Fit and comfort are key, but as base layers fit snugly against the skin, you should pay particular attention to the positioning and thickness of any seams. Look for items that offer flat or 'flat locked' seams, as these will greatly reduce the danger of rubbing. Even better, some manufacturers employ a special 'tubular knit' process that eliminates seams completely.

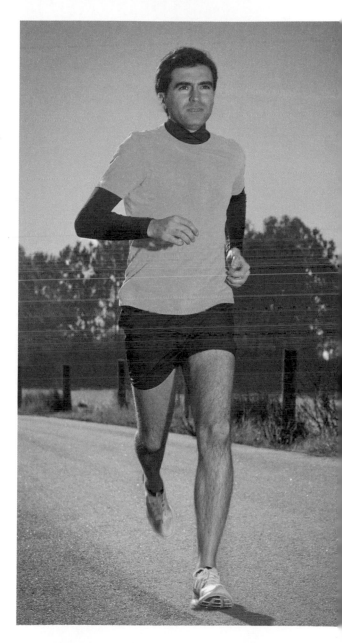

Heat Control

The most expensive base layers offer different levels of thermal properties across different areas of the garment, focusing on the parts that are most likely to lose heat, whilst cutting down in less sensitive areas. Antibacterial properties are also common in base layers – without them, heat and sweat combine to quickly lead to odour.

Hats

The fact that you lose most of your body heat through your head is only true in so far as that tends to be the one part of your body exposed. Finding the right solution to keeping your ears warm is tougher than you might think. Just stick on an old-fashioned woolly hat and you may

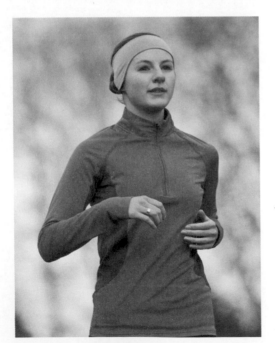

quickly find yourself overheating, even on the coldest of runs. Remember that hats are also vital for keeping the sun off on hot days (see page 68).

Hat Materials

Most running hats have a light fleece lining, which strikes a balance between drawing away sweat and retaining heat. The outer material should be breathable, allowing trapped moisture to escape.

Headbands

When it comes to headwear, keeping it simple is the key. Consider a headband instead of a hat. Headbands keep the vulnerable tips of the ears warm without causing you to overheat. Another good option is a 'tube bandana'. These are seamlessly constructed and designed to be worn in a number of versatile ways – they can be tied into a 'beanie' hat, folded as a headband or slipped down around the neck if your head gets too toasty during the run.

Gloves

As already noted, you will almost always be warmer on a run than you anticipate, but frost-nipped fingers are an occupational hazard. Most gloves designed for running are thinner than normal winter gloves, and come in either natural fibres, such as wool, or synthetics. Wool is a good choice because of its natural ability to regulate heat loss, but wool gloves will get soaked through if you find yourself caught in rain. Synthetic materials – polyesters, acrylics and others – are great when it comes to being weatherproof, but the downside is that they can become sweaty.

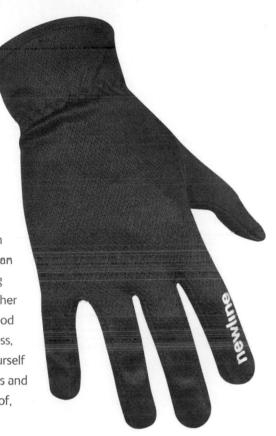

Be Inspired

'One way to keep momentum going is to have constantly greater goals.'
Michael Korda, novelist

How Much to Pay

It is easy enough to pay upwards of £20/$30 for running-specific gloves, but remember that – perhaps more than any other item in your running wardrobe – at some point, you are likely to put them down and lose them. With this in mind, many runners opt for cheap, one-size-fits-all gloves (sometimes sold as 'magic gloves'); there is nothing high-tech about these, but they will do an adequate job whilst minimizing the heartache if you leave them behind at a race.

Jackets

Running jackets come in all shapes and sizes, often with a host of extra features (some useful, many less so), but the key to choosing a jacket is its breathability. If a jacket does not let heat, air and vapour out through its surface, you will quickly feel far too hot.

Jackets add a further layer of insulation, but more important is their function as a wind-stopper. Cold wind blowing against even the best-quality running tops can chill a runner far below the air temperature.

Versatility

Jackets with removable sleeves, to transform them into running gilets, are an excellent idea. Although they often cost more, removable sleeves add to the versatility of this item, and means you can use it nearly all year round.

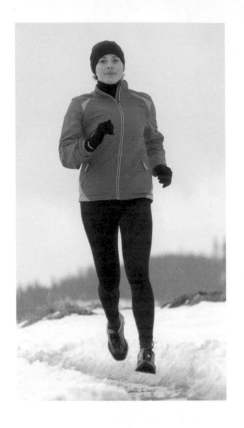

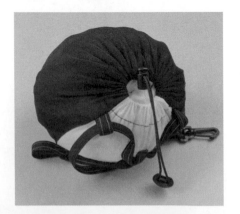

So-called 'micro-jackets' can weigh as little as 80 g (2.8 oz) and can be compressed into their own mesh bag little bigger than a tennis ball. These can be carried on a run just in case, and are also a great option for wearing at the start of a race, when you might be waiting around in cold and windy conditions.

Jackets that compress into a small ball can be very handy as a 'just in case' backup.

Compression Wear

Few, if any, areas of running wear have seen the same rise in popularity in recent years as compression wear. Once the preserve of the elite, this sleek, highly technical-looking race and training apparel has become almost commonplace at even the smallest of local races. For the uninitiated, the choices can be daunting, and phrases such as 'kinesiology-taping technology' do little to encourage runners to part with the not inconsiderable sums of money involved. But there are many benefits to compression wear.

Active or Recovery?

Basically, compression wear is close-fitting apparel designed to hug the muscles tightly, either during exercise or afterwards to speed recovery. Compression wear encompasses everything from socks and tights to T-shirts and long-sleeved tops. Some manufacturers market their compression wear in two distinct categories: race (for training and running) and recovery (post-exercise). In fact, there is little technical difference between the two, so most runners invest only in race compression wear.

What Can Compression Wear Do?

Although some of the claimed benefits of compression wear may seem incredible, most – though not all – have a clear and proven science

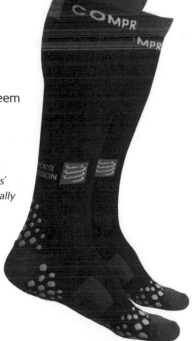

Compressport's 'Full Socks' are designed to be especially effective for recovery.

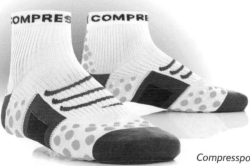

Compressport's 'Pro Racing Socks'

behind them. Firstly, by tightly supporting and gently squeezing certain muscle groups, compression wear will help retain muscle heat, which can both prevent injury and improve performance, particularly over long runs. This 'muscle squeeze' is especially important in compression wear for the legs, as it helps stabilize them and reduce muscle oscillation – the tiny ripples of energy that travel up the legs with each footfall.

Recover Quicker

Another proven benefit is the increased blood flow that well-compressed limbs enjoy. This can maximize performance on the run and speeds up recovery afterwards, significantly reducing leg aches. If you are considering buying compression wear, you are likely to come across the term 'venous return' (sometimes abbreviated to VR). This relates to increased blood flow, but more specifically to blood flow *back* to the heart. Most compression wear uses 'graduated compression' which, for example, changes the amount of squeeze from the ankle and up through the calf, to promote 'venous return'. Some believe that this flushes out lactic acid, but this has not yet been proven.

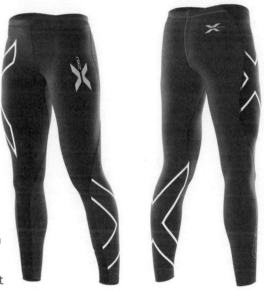

2XU's 'Thermal Compression Tights'

Top Tip

Some runners find full-length recovery tights uncomfortable around the stomach due to post-run 'bloating'. If this happens to you, consider buying compression stockings instead.

Tops Too?

For most runners, a compression T-shirt or top is unlikely to rank high on a list of necessities. There are benefits to these tops – not least the fact that posture and breathing technique may improve – but this specialist clothing can be costly, so invest in the legs first.

Sunglasses

Wearing sunglasses on a bright summer's day might seem like obvious advice, but sunglasses can also be invaluable during winter running, when the sun is low in the sky. As long as they protect fully against the sun's damaging rays (check that they offer 100 per cent UV protection), everyday sunglasses can be fine for running. However, sunglasses designed with the runner in mind offer a wealth of extra benefits.

Comfort is (Almost) Everything

Running sunglasses should be perfectly comfortable; if they're not, you'll soon find yourself discarding a rather expensive investment. There are two keys to comfort: weight and fit.

Weight

The lighter the frame and lens (usually made from high-tech plastic in running sunglasses), the more comfortable they will feel. Ideally, you should hardly notice that you are wearing them, and a sure sign that your sunglasses are too heavy is a 'temple headache', often caused by the weight of the arms on a nerve around the ear.

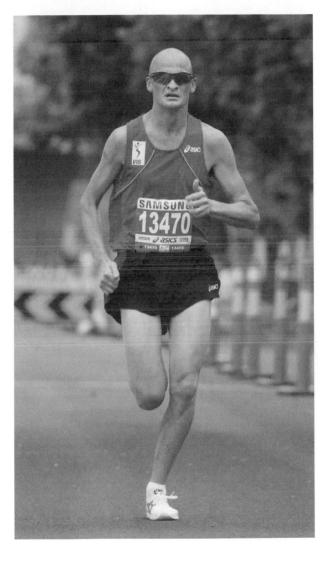

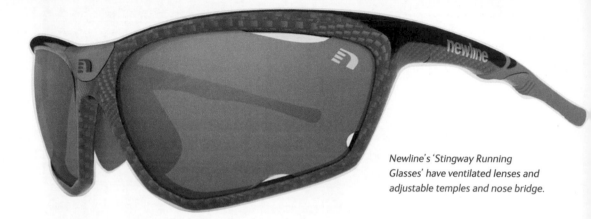

Newline's 'Stingway Running Glasses' have ventilated lenses and adjustable temples and nose bridge.

Fit

When it comes to fit, you need to find a compromise: too giving and your sunglasses will slip down your nose, particularly when you start to sweat; too tight and they can fog up as moisture builds behind the lens. Specialist sports sunglasses address this problem by featuring adjustable elements, such as the nose bridge and the tips of the side arms, as well as by incorporating tiny vents in the frame (sometimes even the lens itself), which prevents them from fogging.

Because fit is so important when choosing the right sunglasses, always try before you buy. If you are making your purchase in a running shop, ask if you can test them out on a treadmill.

Lens Technology

Lens technology has come a long way in the last decade, and there are a number of things to look out for when choosing the right running lenses. As well as those that offer 100 per cent UV protection, running lenses may also be hydrophobic; this simply means that they have

Top Tip

Specialist manufacturers can incorporate prescription lenses into running sunglasses. It's an expensive option, but one that can be worth the investment if your eyesight isn't great.

been treated with a special water-repellent coating to keep off sweat or rain, resulting in a streak-free run, without the hindrance of having to stop and clean your glasses when out and about.

Photochromatic Lenses

Polarized lenses will add considerably to the cost of your sunglasses, but can help virtually eliminate glare. This is useful but not essential for running. Photochromatic lenses (sometimes advertised as 'transitional lenses') are designed to become darker or lighter as lighting conditions change. These are a neat, if expensive, option, but beware of the amount of time that the lenses can take to change – if you run out of bright sunlight and into the relative gloom of some woodland, or even just through an underpass, photochromatic lenses can leave you, literally, in the dark.

Recovery Shoes

It might be enough to slip on a comfortable old pair of slippers after some hard running, but when you

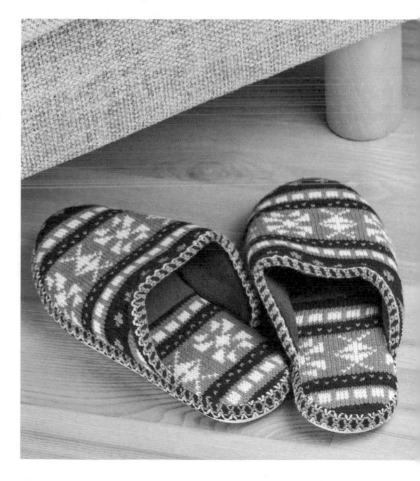

consider that 28 bones, 33 joints and more than 120 muscles and ligaments make up just one foot – all of which will take a hammering during a run – you might like to consider a more scientific approach.

Recovery shoes are not an essential element of a runner's bag of tricks, but with an increasing range on offer – everything from massaging soles to anatomically shaped inserts – anyone prone to post-exercise aching feet might do well to consider them.

Kick Back in Comfort

Comfort is certainly important and, as your feet are likely to swell during a run, it is advisable to choose a pair of recovery shoes that are slightly looser-fitting than regular shoes. Some makes of recovery shoe feature insoles that are specially textured to stimulate blood flow, which speeds post-run recovery. Some take this notion even further, adding hundreds of tiny nodules that are said to activate 'reflex' or acupuncture zones. Although the evidence for this remains controversial, the massaging sensation can still be most welcome.

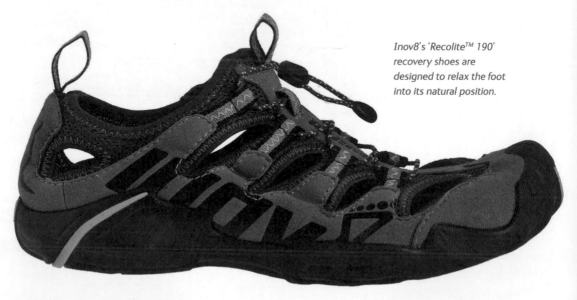

Inov8's 'Recolite™ 190' recovery shoes are designed to relax the foot into its natural position.

Checklist

☑ **Check the material:** Running clothing is made from a huge range of materials, but *always* avoid cotton.

☑ **Safety:** Always look for reflectives incorporated into tops, shorts, tights and even socks.

☑ **Stay cool:** Light colours will keep you cooler on a sunny day.

☑ **Seasonal clothing:** Some clothing can be used for both summer and winter, but check suitability before buying.

☑ **Hitting the trails:** Trail running is a specialist area and requires *some* specialist clothing to maximize comfort and enjoyment.

☑ **Check the temperature:** Too hot or too cold and your run will be miserable. Overestimating cold is common, but try to learn from your mistakes.

☑ **Squeeze it:** Compression wear can be expensive, but can bring a range of benefits for both improving performance *and* speeding recovery.

☑ **Try before you buy:** This is not possible with all clothing, but, whenever you can, put clothing through its paces before making a purchase.

Gadgets

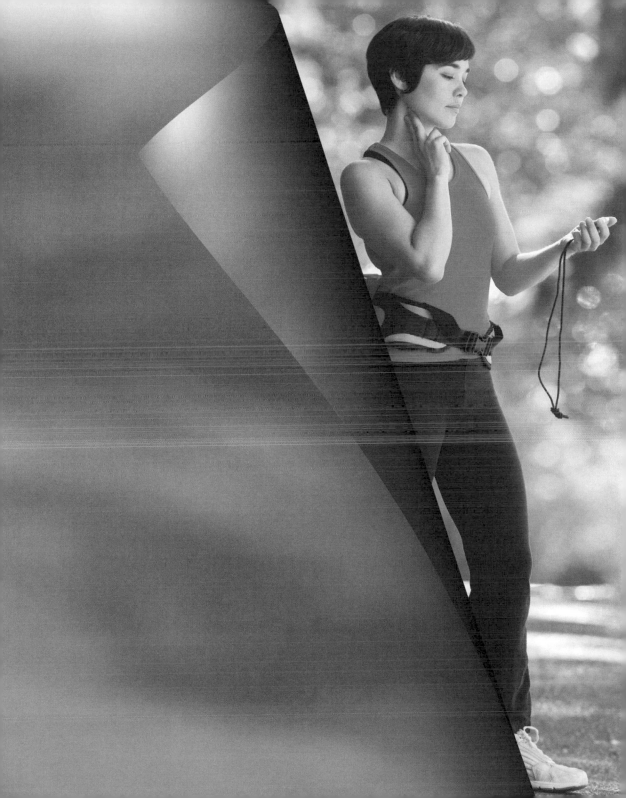

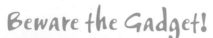

The World of Gadgetry

Once you have your basic running kit – shoes, socks, shorts and a top – you probably think you're good to go. Although those four basic items will get you a long way (indeed they might be all you ever feel you need), there is a whole world of additional running gadgets out there to explore.

Do I Really Need That?

There are some gadgets that you'll find incredibly useful – once purchased, you might even wonder how you ever did without them. However, there is an equal number of running gadgets whose sole purpose seems to be emptying your purse or wallet. Understanding which category your desired gadget falls into can take a little research, as well as some trial and error, but your running needs and goals will determine when and how to spend your money on these extras.

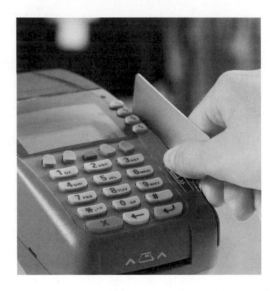

Beware the Gadget!

When it comes to gadgets, things often seem too good to be true. Always bear in mind that this is probably the case, and don't be taken in

Be Inspired

'The only way of finding the limits of the possible is by going beyond them into the impossible.'
Arthur C. Clarke, author

by adverts for the newest health-craze, get-fit-quick gizmo, which promises extraordinary results for minimum effort. Real life seldom works like this.

Be Sceptical

Gadget ads make many promises and claims, but watch out for the following:

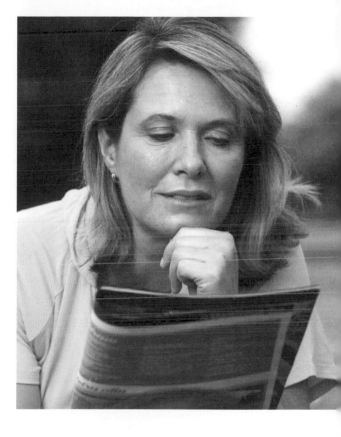

- ☑ **'Expert' testimonials – who are the experts?**
- ☑ **Results of 'research' – who conducted the research?**
- ☑ **Technical or scientific words – look for plain English.**
- ☑ **Statistics – ignore them; you can prove anything with statistics.**
- ☑ **Promises of quick results – worthwhile results take time and effort.**

Top Tip

Online forums are an excellent source of information. If a gadget fails to live up to the hype, forums are the places you'll read about it first.

Although a degree of caution and a dash of healthy scepticism will go a long way in ensuring your money is not squandered, do not be *too* quick to dismiss new gadgets. Once in a while, a revolutionary piece of kit will hit the market in response to new research on training, hydration or nutrition. Not so long ago the idea of a runner strapping a watch capable of being tracked by satellites seemed like the stuff of science fiction, but today they have found their way into millions of runners' lives.

Going the Distance with Gadgets

One of the first additional pieces of kit you might want is something to measure the distances you run. Anything from a basic pedometer costing no more than a few pounds to an all-inclusive Global Positioning System (GPS) watch costing several hundred will do the job, as will a growing number of apps for most makes of smartphone.

Pedometers

A simple pedometer is one of the cheapest and most motivational gadgets that a new runner can invest in. Basic models may cost little more than a few pounds (sometimes they are even given away free with health foods and breakfast cereals). These will do no more than count the number of steps taken, but this is enough to get you started and, with some simple maths, you can calculate the distance you have run.

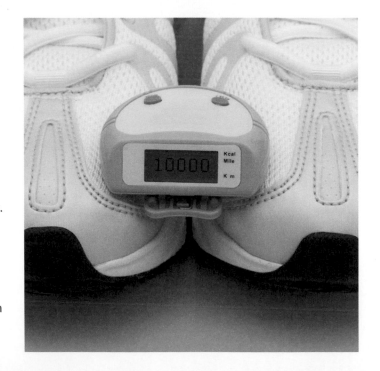

Measuring Distance

Measure a set distance (10 or 20 metres should be enough), then run that distance, counting how many strides it takes. Do this several times and work out the average for greater accuracy. When you use your pedometer on a run, multiply the number of steps it records by your stride length.

Speed or Pace?

'Speed' and 'pace' both describe how fast you are moving. Speed is given as distance per time (e.g. miles per hour). Pace is given as time to travel a distance (e.g. eight-minute mile).

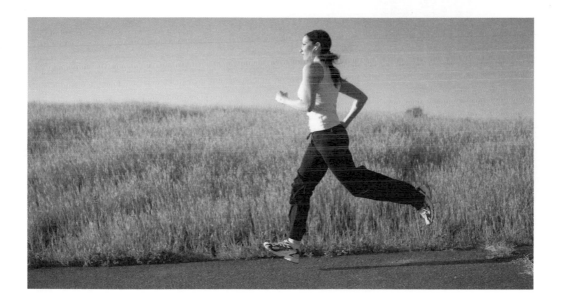

Calibration

One mile is equivalent to approximately 2,000 steps (1,250 steps per kilometre). Your running stride is going to be longer than a regular step, so calibrate your pedometer accordingly. Slightly more expensive pedometers (starting at around £15/$25) will perform the calculations for you to give a distance run, but these will also need to be calibrated when first used, so working out your stride length is still necessary.

Beware of Inaccuracy

Very basic pedometers use a mechanical switch triggered by the movement of a metal ball or tiny pendulum, whilst more advanced and most modern pedometers use a three-way 'inertial sensor', which is more finely tuned and less likely to mis-record movements that are not steps or running strides. Because pedometers use these fairly basic technologies to record the number of steps taken, the level of accuracy is fairly low and the longer the run the greater the inaccuracy. Despite this, they can still be a good starting point for judging how much progress you are making in the comparative distance of your runs.

GPS Watches

There is no denying that a GPS watch is a big investment. Even the most basic model is likely to cost more than your running shoes, and if you adhere to the purity of running – just you and the road – they might seem the reserve of 'gadget junkies'. But, used well, these watches bring an entirely new experience to training harder and running better.

Key features to look for when buying a GPS watch include:

 Weight and comfort   **Reliability of signal**
 Fast satellite connection   **Ease of use**

Top Tip

Look for a GPS watch that connects quickly to the satellite network. 'Acquisition speeds' vary from a few seconds to several minutes.

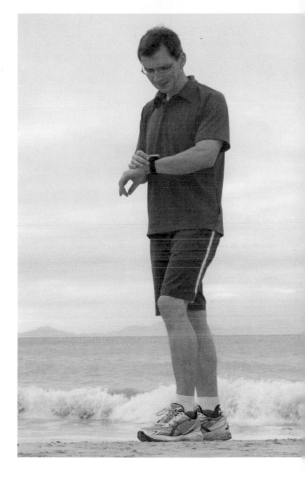

Keeping Track

Just like a car's satellite navigation system, a runner's GPS watch contains a chip-set that communicates with a network of dedicated satellites, using some surprisingly simple mathematics (known as trilateration) to calculate your position – and therefore your speed and distance travelled. Currently, there are 27 GPS satellites orbiting Earth (24 'live' and three backup satellites), at a height of around 19,300 km (12,000 miles). They are arranged so that at any one time there are four in 'line of sight' to you. Most new GPS watches have the chips built into the watch unit, but a few still have a transmitter/receiver that has to be worn separately.

Cost

A basic GPS watch, costing around £120–150/$190–240, will probably only provide fairly basic data – speed, pace and distance. However, as most units use the same (or at least very similar) chip-sets to the most expensive GPS watches, their reliability and accuracy can still be counted on. The majority of chips are made by the same technology giants that dominate the in-car GPS market, so it can be worth looking out for these names – sometimes mentioned in the small print – when shopping.

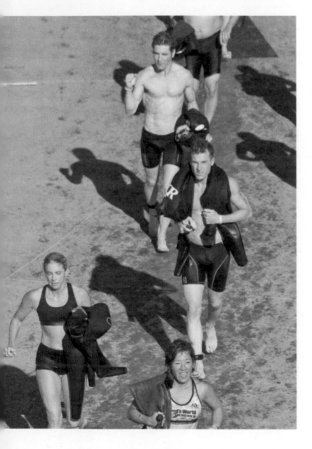

Extra Features

More advanced GPS watches incorporate a host of additional features. Some can record heart rate via a chest strap, although the strap itself is frequently an additional purchase. Others are able to record multi-sports activities, including waterproofing for swimming or ways to calculate accumulative and transition times for triathlons (swim/bike/run). Still others have an optional 'foot pod', which can be used for treadmills when the signal from the satellites isn't available.

Training Partners

One of the most motivational added extras on GPS devices is the Virtual Training Partner (VTP). This is usually an animated icon whose pace is displayed next to your own and which can be set to 'run' at either a predetermined speed – to see how well you are keeping up – or to match your previous best time on the same route. This allows you to measure your improvement.

Online Communities

All good GPS watches come with the ability to connect to a computer (via USB or, increasingly, wirelessly) so that all the data from your run can be uploaded either to the supplied software or to a dedicated website for logging and comparison. A growing number of manufacturers' websites have a range of social networking features, allowing you to share routes, compare results and be inspired by runners in every part of the world. The quality and functions of these websites vary enormously – always take a look at the demo versions before deciding on a brand.

Checklist of GPS Features

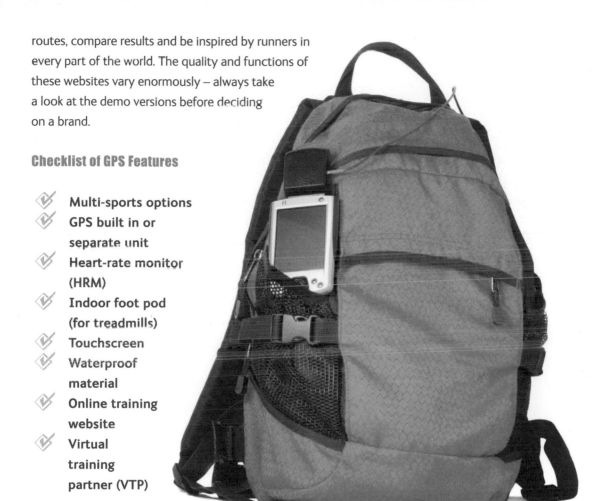

- ☑ **Multi-sports options**
- ☑ **GPS built in or separate unit**
- ☑ **Heart-rate monitor (HRM)**
- ☑ **Indoor foot pod (for treadmills)**
- ☑ **Touchscreen**
- ☑ **Waterproof material**
- ☑ **Online training website**
- ☑ **Virtual training partner (VTP)**

Handheld GPS

Some ultra-distance runners opt for a GPS unit similar to those used for hiking rather than a sports-specific watch version. These can be clipped to a running backpack, are more rugged and better waterproofed, and also have the advantage of changeable batteries rather than relying on recharging via a computer.

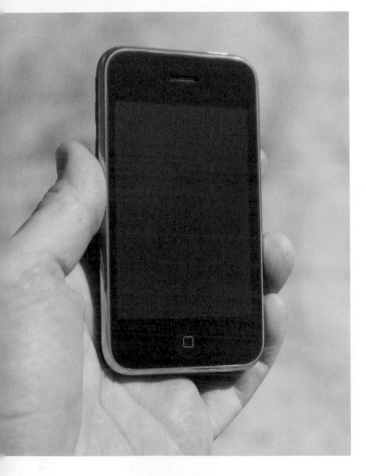

Going Mobile

Modern smartphones do far more than just make calls. With inbuilt GPS and a range of apps on offer, using your phone as a training aid is an increasingly popular and infinitely cheaper option than investing in a dedicated GPS watch.

Running Apps

Many apps cost as little as £2/$2 and will generally display and record basic information such as location, pace, distance and time, as well as including access to a social networking-style site for logging and sharing your runs. Because smartphone straps/holders for running are usually attached to the upper arm (as opposed to the wrist mount of a GPS watch), they can be difficult to see and operate, and touch-screen functions can be tricky to use – virtually impossible with gloves.

What to look for in an app:

 No adverts

 Ease of use – a simple start/stop button is best

 Clear, easily read data

 Support website with social networking

Top Tip

Free apps can be cluttered with adverts, making an already crowded smartphone screen difficult to decipher. Paying for an ad-free app is worth it.

Gadgets for Staying Safe

Absolutely nothing is more important than your safety whilst running. If you spend your money on nothing else, spend it ensuring that you are seen and safe. Basic safety gadgets – something as simple as a snap-on reflective cuff – cost very little and can be life-savers. Almost all running gear is now available with inbuilt reflective or high-visibility detailing, but don't stop there – the more reflectives and lights, the better. No one was ever injured by being too visible.

Reflectivity

Running at night and in poor weather conditions needs great attention to safety. Modern reflective materials are incredibly light and relatively inexpensive, so there is no excuse for not adding them to your general running kit. There is a range of patented materials, but 3M™ Scotchlite is one of the most common. Whatever material your gear is made from, always check the advertised specifications, which state an approximate distance at which visibility is provided. Always go for the maximum.

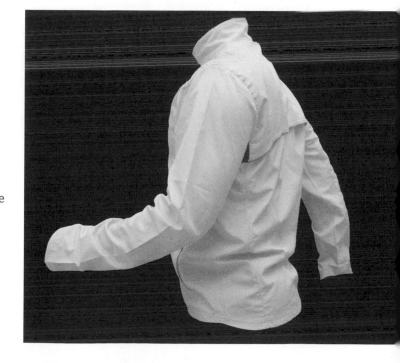

Integrated Reflectives

Many items of running clothing include integrated reflective strips or logos. Even if you're choosing a top for summer running, there is no harm in finding one that includes safety detailing, as this will extend its usefulness year round. Running jackets almost always include high-visibility patches, but make sure they offer 360-degree visibility – meaning they will reflect light from the front, back and sides. Fluorescent or reflective headbands are an excellent way of adding to 360-degree visibility.

When choosing clothing for its safety features, always look carefully to see exactly how much reflective detailing is included. Sometimes it can be as little as a tag or strip on the cuff, which is not nearly enough.

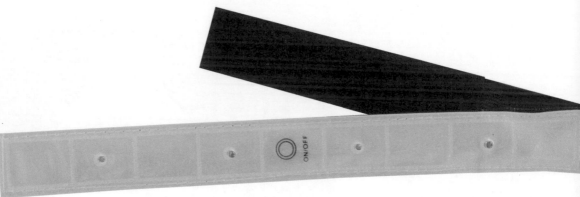

This armband is doubly effective, with blinking lights as well as reflective material.

Armbands and Sashes

Add reflectivity to your running kit with simple armbands or a sash similar to those worn by many cyclists. Both items are amongst the least expensive and most important things a runner can own. Look for an armband that fits securely and will not slip down your arm; Velcro is great, but an increasing number of 'snap bands' are now available, which lock when snapped around the arm.

Lights

A growing range of safety gear is available with light-emitting diode (LED) technology built into it. Some reflective armbands add a greater degree of visibility by including these tiny lightweight bulbs, usually with a flashing 'strobe' mode. You can even buy running hats with integrated lights. The disadvantage of lights over simple reflectives is that they require batteries, which could run down at the most inconvenient or critical time.

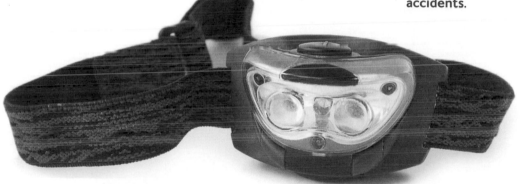

Head Torches

A head torch will not only add to your safety, but will help illuminate the road ahead. Most modern head torches – ranging in price from £20/$30 to an eye-watering £200/$300-plus – employ small, lightweight and long-lasting LED technology.

Torch Weight

When choosing a head torch, make sure that it is as light and comfortable as possible. Try before you buy and use a little jogging on the spot to make sure that there is not too much bounce. Remember that a shop model is unlikely to already have batteries fitted, so account for this extra weight when testing; battery weight can add significantly to the bulk, and models that take four or more batteries, even at AAA size, can feel cumbersome.

Going the Distance

Check the 'burn time' advertised for the head torch. This refers to how long a single set of batteries should last, but be aware that the time given is probably how long the batteries will last under *ideal* conditions – something you are unlikely to find in the real world, where extreme temperatures have a dramatic impact on burn time. More expensive head torches will feature a variety of modes, including flashing/strobe, but using these modes will also reduce the battery life.

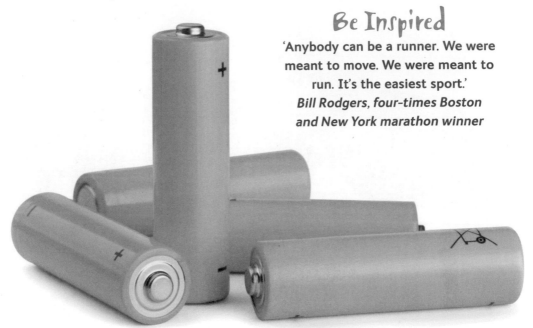

Be Inspired

'Anybody can be a runner. We were meant to move. We were meant to run. It's the easiest sport.'
Bill Rodgers, four-times Boston and New York marathon winner

Many Candles

Just as with cycling lights, the brightness of a head torch is often given in a bewildering array of measurements, including 'candles', 'lumens' and 'cendelas'. It is simpler to look for how many LEDs are built in (anything from one to 10 or more) – the more LEDs, the more light it will provide. Remember, though, that the greater the number, the shorter the life expectancy of the batteries is likely to be.

The Healthy Gizmo Guide

Using the term 'gadget' seems a little frivolous when it comes to matters of health. However, there are many items on the market that purport to be for the good of your health but, in fact, will do little more than provide you with another set of numbers to log. On the other hand, some additional kit can be extremely useful in helping you both train and run much more efficiently.

Heart Rate Monitors

Few running gadgets divide people as fiercely as HRMs. Some see them as an unnecessary technology 'ballast' that clutters a good run and simply provides too much information, whilst others swear by them as a way of monitoring both fitness and progression. The choice is personal, but a greater understanding of how they can be used may help you make up your mind.

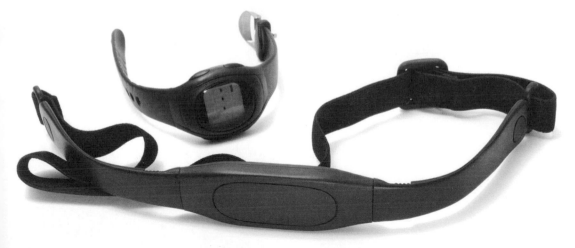

Cost and Features

HRMs range in price from as little as £20/$30 to more than £100/$160. The most basic ones come in two pieces: a strap or belt that secures around the chest and measures the heart rate, and a wrist-mounted watch that receives the data wirelessly and provides a readout of beats per minute. Although all HRMs combine other basic information such as elapsed time on the run, more expensive models can calculate and display other variables, including what percentage of your run is spent in a particular 'heart-rate zone', and feeding back a combination of visual and audio alarms as the zones change.

Be Inspired

'It does not matter how slowly you go, so long as you do not stop.'
Confucius, philosopher

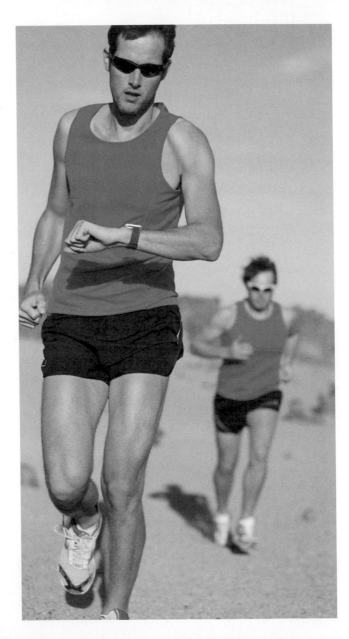

Staying in the Zone

Heart-rate zones are calculated as percentages of your maximum heart rate (MHR). Running in these different zones (basically at different speeds) will have different training results.

 Energy efficient zone:
With an HRM showing your heart beating at around 60–70 per cent of its maximum, you should be building your endurance (long-run) capabilities. This is also the zone that works best for fat-burning (weight loss), and should set the pace for both the warming up start of a run and the cooling down final section.

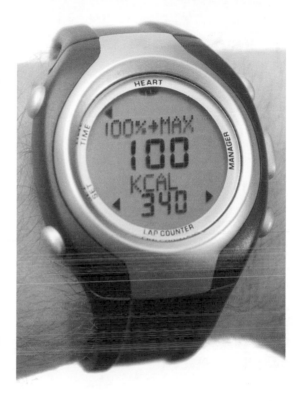

 The aerobic zone: At 70–80 per cent of maximum heart rate, you will be in the aerobic zone, which helps develop your cardiovascular system (heart and blood supply). Fat-burning continues in this zone and, as your fitness improves, more of your run may be spent at this level.

 The anaerobic zone: At 80–90 per cent of maximum heart rate, fat-burning is massively reduced and your body is likely to be using more energy stored in the muscles. This can lead to lactic acid build-up, which causes fatigue.

Estimate Your Maximum Heart Rate

MHR = 206 − (0.7 × age)

Sprint zone: 90–100 per cent of maximum effort is reserved for sprint finishes and for short bursts of running for interval training.

Blood-pressure Monitors

Blood-pressure monitors, technically known as sphygmomanometers, were once the preserve of the medical profession, but, in recent years, a dramatic fall in price has led to many basic units – costing as little as £15/$25 – being readily available on the high street.

Avoid BP Obsession

It is true that blood pressure is an excellent indicator of overall health, but there is a danger in owning your own unit – it's easy to become obsessed with checking results on an almost daily basis. Unless there is a medical need to constantly monitor your own blood pressure, there is little point in investing even a small amount of your own money on a blood-pressure monitor.

Massage Gadgets

Massaging tired feet and legs is not only a relaxing and rewarding post-run activity, but it can help to improve blood flow too, which speeds the recovery process. It also helps loosen tight and exhausted muscles. It is possible to self-massage with nothing more than your hands – perhaps with the addition of mild massage oil or cream – but to really work the magic, it might be worth investing in a massage ball or roller.

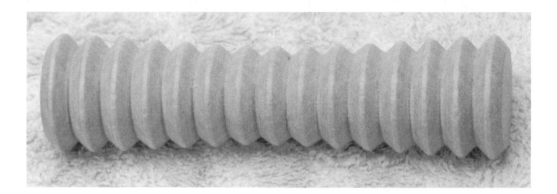

Ribbed Rollers

This is probably the simplest massage gadget available – and certainly the cheapest. A ribbed roller is simply a textured tube that can be placed under the foot and rolled backwards and forwards. Pressure can be varied just by pressing harder or more gently, and the simple to and-fro motion quickly revives tired feet and stimulates the flow of blood. Look for wooden rather than plastic models, as they have a more pleasing feel against bare skin.

Ball Massagers

These come in two varieties: dimpled and smooth. Smooth ball massagers are usually housed in a plastic collar with bearings to help them glide more easily. Because they are more technically engineered, expect to pay between £10/$15 and £20/$30. Dimpled ball massagers are cheaper, and have the advantage of stimulating blood flow, although the sensation can take some getting used to. All ball-style massagers can be used on the whole body in addition to working wonders on the feet.

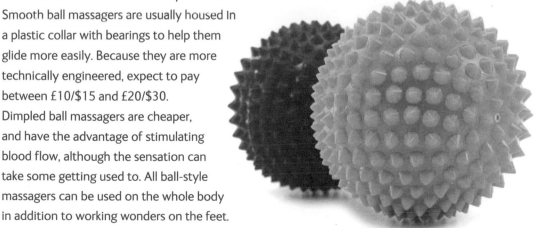

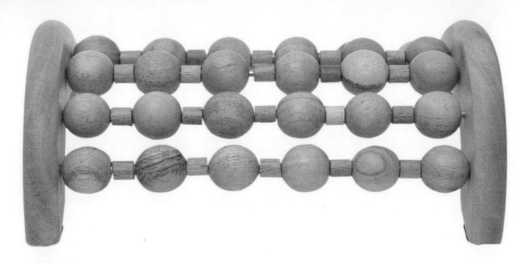

Bead Massagers

These are designed specifically for the feet, with rows of beads arranged on a frame that can be placed flat on the ground as you move your foot across it. Wooden varieties tend to be harder-wearing and feel better underfoot than plastic. This style of massage requires very little effort, and is perfect for some simple pampering whilst reading or watching television. Expect to pay in the region of £10/$15.

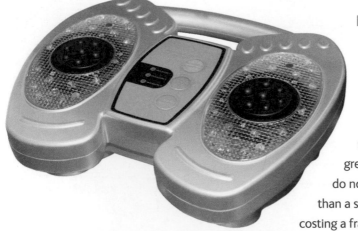

High-tech Solutions

High-tech massagers can cost as much as £100/$160. They offer many additional features, such as various vibration speeds and even heat settings. They are undoubtedly a great treat, but health-wise, they do not offer any greater advantage than a simple massage roller or ball costing a fraction of the price.

Music Players

Not all running gadgets can be considered truly *useful*, but there are plenty that can enliven training. Listening to music on a run – when it is safe to do so – can be incredibly motivating, and sports MP3 players and playlists designed for runners are now a massive market. Today's MP3 players are so small and light that there's no excuse for leaving your music at home.

Safety First

When it comes to using MP3 players, safety cannot be emphasized strongly enough. You should only ever listen to music on routes you know to be safe and traffic-free – and even then, they should only be set at volumes low enough to hear a shouted warning. Many organized events and races ban the use of MP3 players; always adhere to race rules – they are not imposed to spoil your fun but rather for both your own and other competitors' safety. It is crucial to clearly hear warnings or instructions from race marshals, even on off-road sections that might otherwise seem safe.

Choosing the Right Player

Many MP3 players are designed specifically for sports; these tend to be more rugged and weatherproof, but also more expensive. In fact, most regular MP3 players should be more than up to the job of entertaining you on a run; just be aware that you'll need to protect them from the elements and choose a player with easy-to-operate buttons and menus. It can be worth buying a truly budget model and saving more expensive and technical players from the rigours of a run entirely.

MP3 Holders

The majority of MP3 players are now small enough to fit into even the smallest pockets on your running shorts, but a dedicated holder, which straps the player to the upper arm, can be very useful for easy access. Look for a holder that fastens securely – Velcro is ideal – so that the MP3 player stays firmly in place. Also check how much weatherproofing is incorporated.

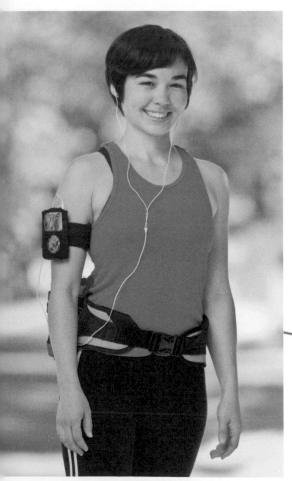

Earphones

Specialist running earphones are expensive and largely unnecessary. Just select earphones that are light and comfortable and, most importantly, stay in the ear. Some earphones include inline volume-control buttons that override an MP3 player's controls, which is useful for quick volume changes.

Top Tip

Touch-screen players can be fiddly to operate whilst running (virtually impossible in gloves), so choose a player with large, obvious buttons.

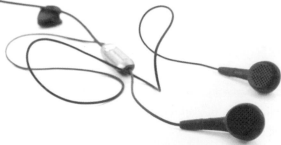

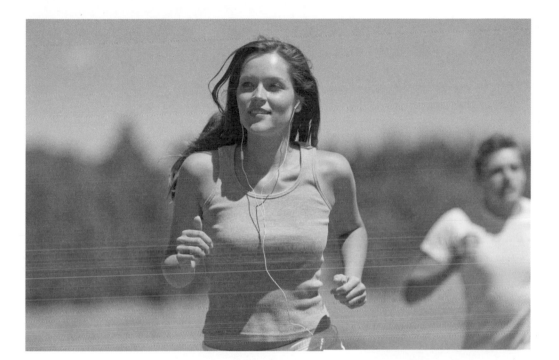

Creating a Playlist

There are almost as many types of running as there are genres of music and, although a growing number of commercial running playlist albums are available, nothing beats putting together your own collection of favourite tracks to match the mood.

Top Tip

Make three or more playlists of songs with similar beats, so that you can switch between them as your mood and pace change.

Fast or Slow?

It may seem obvious, but faster running suits faster tracks and slower running, perhaps plodding up hills, best suits slower tracks. As a general rule, a track with 120 beats per minute or fewer is well suited to the start of a run, whilst picking up your pace will require a faster track, with 165 beats or more per minute.

Gadgets for Going Further

As your running improves and you begin to go for longer distances, a few additional gadgets will become increasingly important. Any run longer than an hour or so is going to require hydration. This means water, which in turn means you need a way of carrying a water bottle. This might seem straightforward, but the array of bottles available can be bewildering. Similarly, ways of carrying running gels and bars for half-marathons and marathons are amazingly diverse, and when it comes to backpacks there is also a multitude of options.

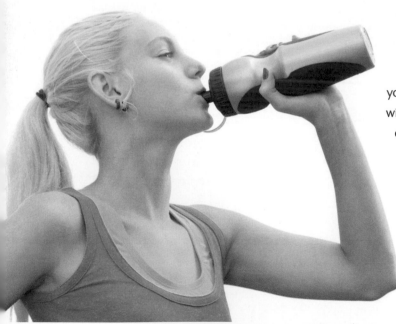

Hydration Solutions

At some point on your journey to becoming a fully fledged runner, you'll need to carry a supply of water with you. Unless the conditions are extremely hot, this is likely to be at the point when you are running for an hour or more.

Be Inspired

'I failed my way to success.'
Thomas Edison, inventor

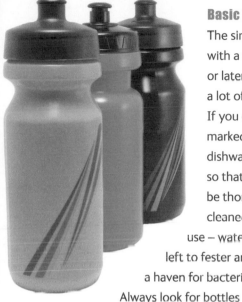

Basic Bottles

The simplest water bottles are tough but lightweight plastic with a typical capacity of 500 ml. Enter a few races and sooner or later a free one will turn up in your finishers' prize bag; enter a lot of races and you'll find you accrue quite a few of these. If you do need to buy a water bottle, look for ones that are marked as being dishwasher safe, so that they can be thoroughly cleaned after use – water bottles left to fester are a haven for bacteria. Always look for bottles marked 'BPA-free' – BPA (bisphenol A) is a compound found in older bottles, or some cheaper imported bottles, and is believed to have adverse health effects.

Ergonomic Bottles

Because a regular bottle can be difficult to grip on the run – particularly in sweaty hands or with gloves – many bottles are contoured for an ergonomic grip. Fancier ones are constructed in an elongated loop design, in which the water fills the handle as well as the bottle. These are often available in smaller capacities, generally 250–300 ml, and can be excellent for shorter runs in hot weather.

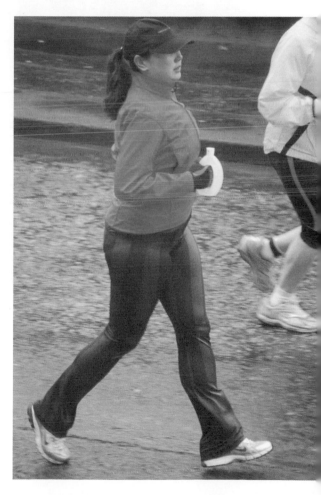

Straw Designs

Bottles with flip tops and integrated straws that draw water up from the bottom of the bottle make it unnecessary to have to tip the bottle to drink. They are usually intended for use with running backpacks, which are designed to fit one (sometimes two) bottles in loops or pockets built into the straps. This more technical design adds to the overall weight of the bottle.

Bladders

Soft, flexible bladders are designed for use in specialist running backpacks or belts. They offer several advantages over bottles that need to be carried by hand. Generally they have a larger capacity (2 litres or more), making them best suited for longer runs such as marathons, or for extended trail and adventure running.

Because they are flexible, they mould to the contours of the hips or back for maximum comfort. Integrated 'feed tubes', which can be clipped to a running top, mean that water is always at hand (or mouth), and this encourages more frequent hydration. Look for a bladder that incorporates an antibacterial compound to ensure that the water you carry is always safe to drink.

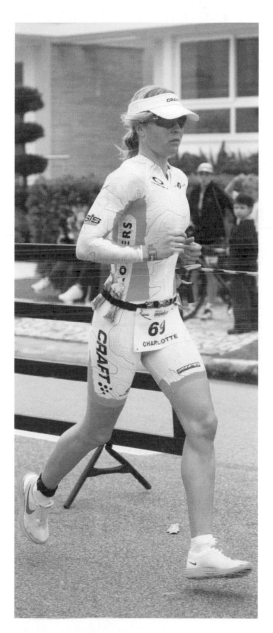

Carrying Gels and Bars

With longer runs comes the need for nutrition as well as hydration, and in most practical terms this means gels, bars or similar running snacks. A run of up to 90 minutes will probably require little more than a single gel (in which case, a small pocket in your shorts or shirt will be adequate), but half-marathons and beyond will certainly need multiple gels and bars.

Top Tip

Carefully wash out the bladder after use, then store it in a freezer to prevent the build-up of bacteria. Remember to thaw fully before using.

Keep It Simple

One of the best solutions for carrying gels and bars is an elasticated race belt. This comprises little more than a double twist of elasticated material, which secures around the waist and allows the gels to be tucked through the loops of fabric. These belts weigh next to nothing and can cost as little as £5/$8. Some feature a small extra zip pocket for storing keys.

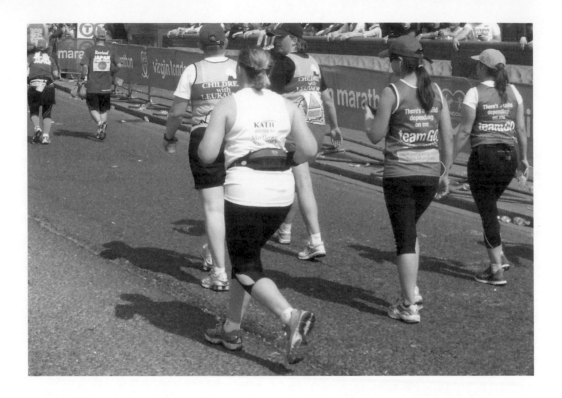

Bum Bags

If you opt for a bum bag (a.k.a. fanny pack) to carry your running snacks, look for a sports-specific make. These will cost around £25/$40, but they are low-profile – designed to sit close to the back to minimize bouncing, which can become unbearable over time. Weight is important, but look to balance this with some degree of padding on the side that will be pressed against your back/bottom. Choose a bum bag that fits just the number of gels you need – excess space leads to a temptation to overfill with things you almost certainly will not need.

Top Tip

Backpacks and bum bags are likely to be worn for long periods. Always try before you buy – ideally test a friend's pack and really put it through its paces.

Pre-loaded Belts

Running magazines are often awash with adverts for running belts that come complete with a range of energy gels, recovery bars and other sports-nutrition products designed to get you through a marathon. Unless you are absolutely sure that these are products you know and like, they are best avoided. Every runner has different needs and tastes, so a one-solution-fits-all belt is unlikely to be value for money.

Backpacks

Running with a backpack might seem to be going against the purity of stripped-down exercise, but there are many good reasons to consider one. Running to and from work is becoming increasingly popular as a way to stay fit whilst avoiding high travel costs and time wasted in congestion. And as your running distances increase, you may want to carry more kit with you.

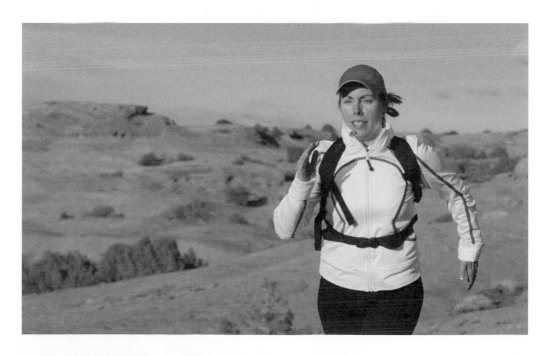

Specialist Sports Packs

Although considerably more expensive than normal backpacks or rucksacks (around £60–150/ $90–240), sports packs are specifically designed to be comfortable, durable and to have weight distribution that takes the motion of running into account. Make sure that the straps are flat and comfortable, and if they have a larger capacity – and are thus likely to be heavier when fully loaded – ensure that they incorporate a chest (or sternum) strap to take some of the load away from the shoulders and hips. Never be tempted to overload a backpack – neck, shoulder and back problems can result from excessive weight. A variety of other features may be included, but chief amongst these should be reflective visibility strips on both the back and front straps.

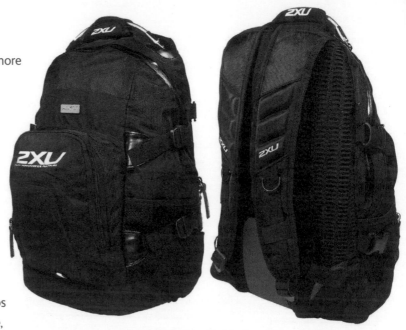

2XU's 25-litre Backpack

Water for Packs

Most running packs will either incorporate a water bladder or have somewhere to store a bottle. Check that your water will be easily accessible; water carried but not drunk is dead weight and dehydration can be dangerous.

Top Tip

Female-specific backpacks are available, generally with a shorter length and ergonomically designed for a smaller frame.

Checklist

✓ **Need vs. want:** How worthwhile is the latest gadget? Make sure your money is well spent and avoid buying something that just looks good.

✓ **Check the evidence:** What scientific proof does the latest gizmo offer for improving your running or health?

✓ **Count the cost:** If all you want to know is how far you have run, a simple pedometer might win out over an expensive GPS device.

✓ **GPS needs:** Check which goals you have set. Which additional GPS features will measure your improvements or aid your training?

✓ **Safety:** How much safety kit do you have? There is no such thing as too much visibility.

✓ **Get in the zone:** Do you need to measure your heart rate? If you want to work 'in the zone', an HRM is essential.

✓ **Sound advice:** Is your route safe for listening to music?

✓ **Stay hydrated:** Make sure you can safely and comfortably carry enough water for a run. Consider the wide range of hydration solutions carefully.

✓ **Pack fit:** From bum bags to full race packs, make sure you can comfortably carry all your food and water, but never overload yourself when setting off for a run.

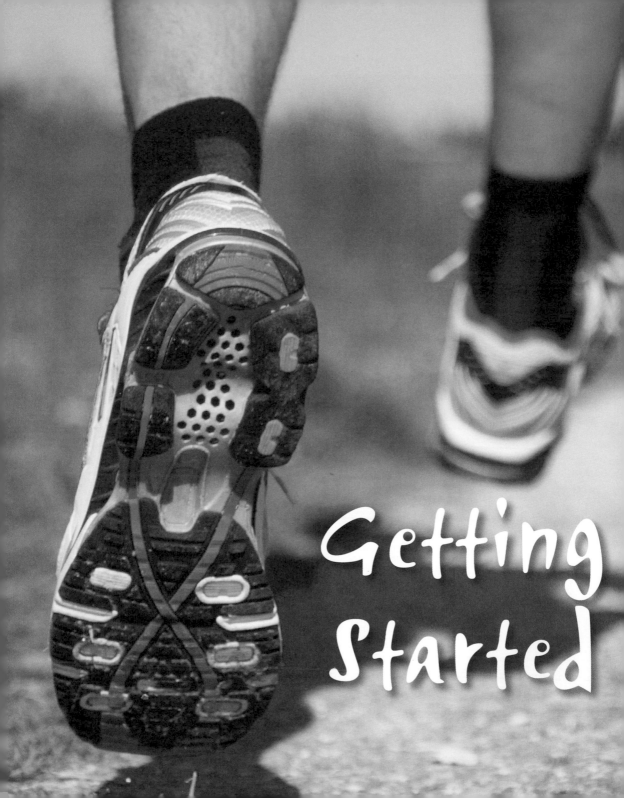

Getting Started

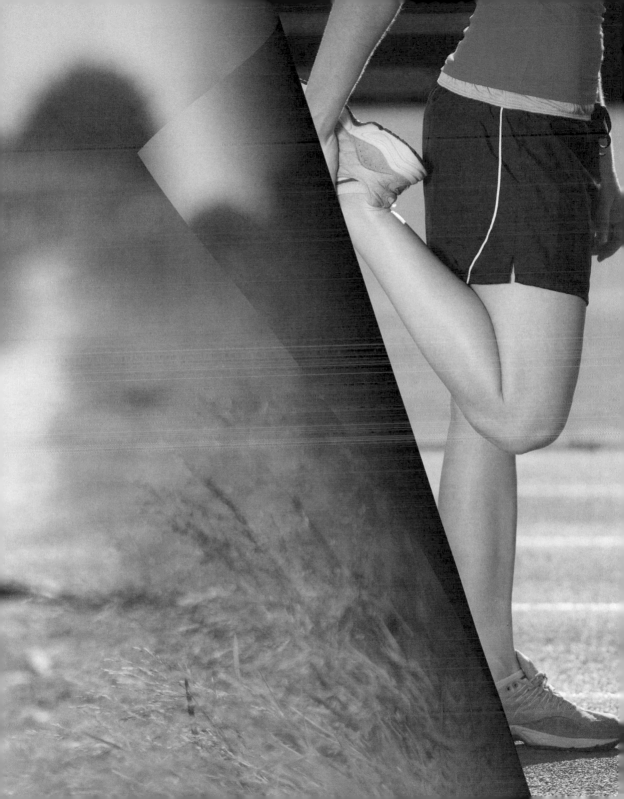

Weights and Measures

'Oh, I could never run!' This is a refrain you have probably heard frequently, or even uttered yourself. Once you are a fully fledged runner, you will just as often hear people telling you, hopefully with a touch of admiration, 'I could *never* do what you do'. But the simple truth is that most of us *can* – and probably should.

Am I Fit Enough to Run?

The usual answer is yes! With the exception of certain medical conditions and illnesses, there are few reasons not to run. In fact, there are many health benefits in hitting the streets and trails. If in doubt, always seek medical advice before you take up running. It is also worth taking the time before you start to set a few benchmarks against which you can measure your progress.

Check Your Blood Pressure

A runner's blood pressure (BP) is usually considerably lower than that of non-runners. Most gyms and many doctors' surgeries have a blood-pressure monitor (or sphygmomanometer), and they are usually self-service so you won't need to make an appointment to get a reading.

The monitor will return a result that looks something like 125/90, usually expressed as '125 over 90'. The first number is the 'systolic value' – the pressure as the heart beats, forcing the flow of blood. The second reading is known as the 'diastolic value' – effectively the pressure of the heart as it 'relaxes' between beats.

Understanding Your Reading

Blood-pressure ranges can broadly be defined as follows:

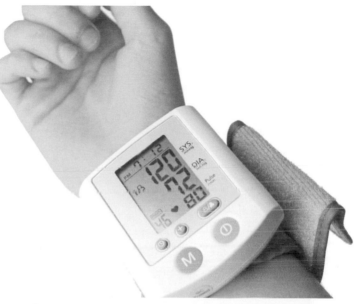

- ☑ **Over 120/80 – steps should be taken to lower BP**
- ☑ **Under 120/80 – ideal for a healthy lifestyle**
- ☑ **105/65 – elite runner's BP**

Heart Rate

Measuring your resting heart rate is one of the quickest and most reliable ways of determining your starting fitness. This is simply your heart rate taken at a time when you are not (and have not been) exercising.

Top Tip

As it can be affected by many external factors, always seek professional medical advice if you have any concerns about your blood pressure.

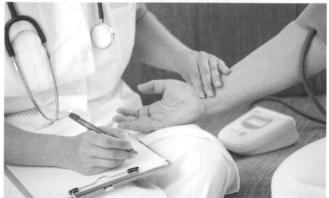

Measuring Heart Rate

For greatest accuracy, measure your heart rate as soon as you wake in the morning. Touch the middle and index finger of one hand against the base of the thumb on the wrist of the other hand, and count the beats for one minute. Taking an average reading over several days will give you a more accurate count. Heart rate is given as beats per minute (BPM).

Heart-rate Ranges

Heart-rate ranges can be broadly defined as follows:

- ✅ **30–50 BPM – elite athlete**
- ✅ **50–70 BPM – running fit**
- ✅ **70–80 BPM – average rate**
- ✅ **80–100 BPM – unfit**

Body Mass Index

Your body mass index (BMI) is an indication of how over- or underweight you are, and is calculated using your height-to-weight ratio.

Calculating BMI

To calculate your own BMI, weigh yourself in pounds and multiply by 703, then divide the figure by your height in inches squared. If that all seems too complex, there are many online calculators that will work this out for you.

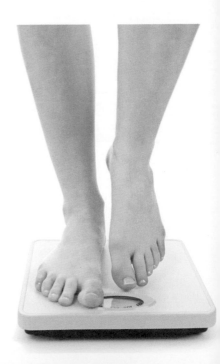

A BMI of 25 or more indicates that you are overweight; 18.5 or less suggests you are underweight. However, this method does not distinguish between weight from muscle and weight from fat, which means that a perfectly healthy but particularly muscular athlete could register as obese on this scale. For this reason, many doctors (and runners) look instead to body fat index.

Body Fat Index

The body fat index (BFI) is calculated using a precision reader, which can be found in most gyms and doctors' surgeries. The results are more accurate than the ready-reckoner of BMI and, because it can distinguish between muscle and fat, BFI is a better overall indicator of health and is a useful benchmark figure to know when taking up running.

Average BFIs

The healthy BFI range for a man is different to that of a woman. The average man has 15–17 per cent body fat, the average woman 18–22 per cent. Values for elite athletes are 6–12 per cent for men and 12–20 per cent for women.

Be Inspired

'Don't be afraid to give up the good to go for the great.'
John D. Rockefeller, philanthropist

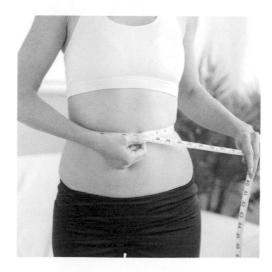

Waist to Hip Ratio

Knowing your waist-to-hip ratio (WHR) can also be a useful starting figure against which to gauge your progress. Relax your stomach and measure the narrowest part of your waist, then measure the widest point of your hips. Divide your waist measurement by your hip measurement. A figure of one or less for a man and 0.85 or less for a woman is desirable.

Weight Issues

Many people take up running to help with weight loss, and medical evidence suggests that 50 per cent more calories are burned when running compared to walking. But certain precautions should be taken by runners carrying excessive weight:

- Consult your doctor for advice on how best to combine running and diet.
- Never mix 'crash' or 'detox' diets with running; your body needs fuel!
- Keep both pace and distance low to avoid common stress injuries.
- Take a water bottle even on the shortest run; overweight runners sweat more.
- Chafing and rubbing can be a problem – use Vaseline or anti-chafe creams.
- Replace running shoes regularly – greater weight equals greater wear.
- Keep clothing loose and comfortable.

Too Old to Run?

Age is rarely a barrier to running. It is true that speed can decrease with age, which is why marathons and other distance runs are increasingly full of runners in their fifties, sixties, seventies and beyond. With age often comes greater determination and mental stamina, so there are no barriers to taking up running even later in life, as long as you take a sensible approach to training, including ensuring that you rest properly and recover. In 2011, at the age of 100, Fauja Singh became the world's oldest marathon runner when he completed the Toronto Waterfront Marathon. He was 89 when he took up running.

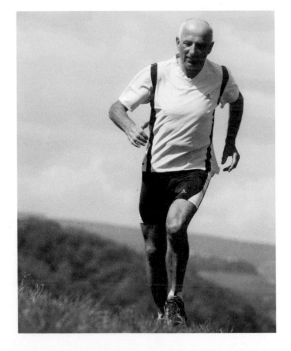

Age Concerns

Despite this, older runners should be aware of several possible issues.

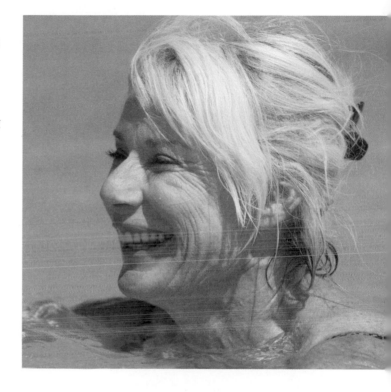

- **Vulnerable bones:** Bone density falls with age, making some common running injuries (particularly stress fractures) more likely. Switch speed for distance and increase workouts gradually.

- **Slower recovery:** Due to a combination of factors, including changes to the muscle fibres, recovery takes longer as you age. Take time to recover and heal.

- **Degenerative disorders:** Conditions such as osteoarthritis are more common in older runners; keep your weight down to counteract the risk of injury.

- **Flexibility:** General flexibility decreases with age, so add some cross training, swimming and even yoga to help balance things out.

- **Slowing heart rate:** Maximum heart rate reduces with age (by about one beat a year); maintain a general healthy lifestyle and diet to help your running.

Be Inspired
'**Human beings are made up of flesh and blood, and a miracle fibre called courage.**'
George Patton, US general.

Kids Run Too

Of course kids can run too – as a natural part of outdoor play children can run around for hours. However, when it comes to focused, goal-orientated training, a more measured approach needs to be taken.

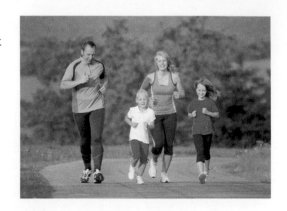

Team Games

Children under the age of 10 have a more limited capacity for endurance. General fitness is therefore better targeted through a combination of speed, co-ordination and flexibility, which makes team sports such as football, hockey and netball so popular.

Family Runs

Many organized running events for adults include family and fun runs, especially designed to get children involved at an early age. These can be a great way of getting the whole family engaged and interested in your favourite pastime, and can go a long way to preventing any resentment your kids might feel at the time and effort you spend training.

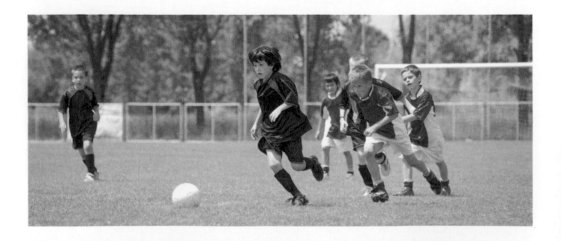

Kit for Kids

Just as all adult runners need specialist running kit, so do children. Shorts and tops should be designed for running (never made of cotton). Shoes should be fitted properly and checked regularly against the growth of the feet – running in generic trainers can do long-lasting, even permanent, damage. Do not despair about cost, though: many high-street sports shops have reasonably priced running kit designed for children.

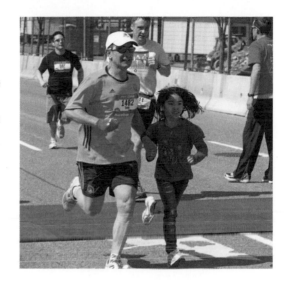

Pregnancy

Few doctors are likely to suggest that you take up running once pregnant, but if you are already a runner there is little reason to stop running until you are well into pregnancy. Do listen to your body, though, and don't push distance or pace. Hydration is vital and you may find yourself needing more water than usual on a run. Later in pregnancy, your centre of gravity will begin to shift as your bump grows, and this – combined with looser and weaker joints – can increase the risk of injuries such as twisted ankles, runner's knee and Achilles tendonitis. *Consult your doctor or health visitor about any concerns you may have.*

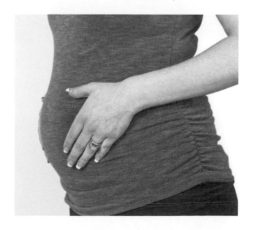

Top Tip

Encourage your children to take an interest in your running. Some events even allow them to run to the finish line with you!

Post-natal Running

There are plenty of reasons to continue running after childbirth. Beyond the obvious health benefits, post-natal running also offers an opportunity to get out of the house at a time when cabin fever might be setting in. Many gyms and running clubs arrange organized buggy-jogging sessions, where new mums can run with their pushchairs along safe, accessible routes.

Buggy Runs

If you're out running with your child in a buggy, follow these tips.

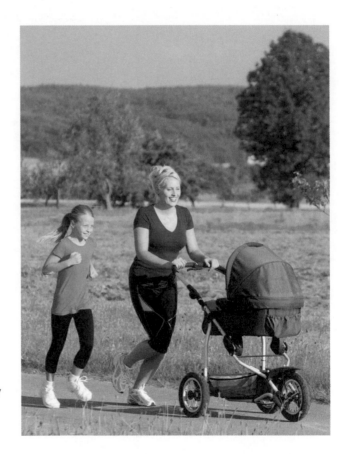

- ☑ **Keep it level**: Stick to flat, smooth-surfaced routes.

- ☑ **Stay away from traffic**: Avoid heavily congested roads with greater pollution.

- ☑ **Stay safe**: Run with friends or in a group.

- ☑ **Short runs**: Even the most patient baby is likely to get bored eventually; keep runs short.

- ☑ **Save money**: Most buggies are suitable for gentle running, so do not waste money on expensive 'sports' models.

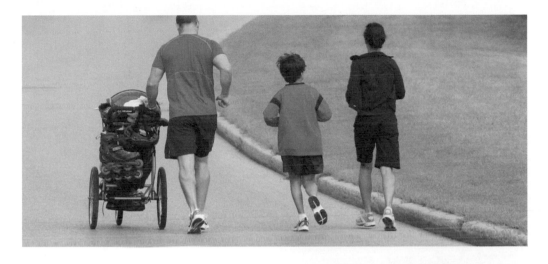

✅ **Relax**: Try pushing with one hand so the other swings naturally; switch hands frequently.

✅ **Warm and happy**: Make sure your child is warm – they will feel the cold even when you do not.

✅ **Avoid baby slings**: Never run with a papoose-style carrier, as bad running posture can lead to back and neck injuries.

Be Inspired
'Ask yourself: "Can I give more?" The answer is usually: "Yes."'
Paul Tergat, marathon runner

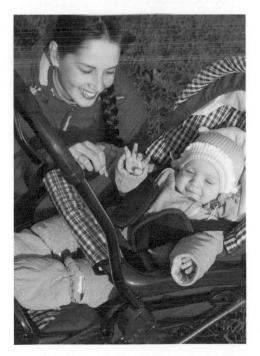

Becoming a Runner

Running freely and with great pleasure is something we all did as children, but as time passes many of us lose the confidence to just go for it. Starting to run again as an adult – whatever the initial motivation – is all about recapturing the uncomplicated joy of putting one foot in front of the other in rapid succession.

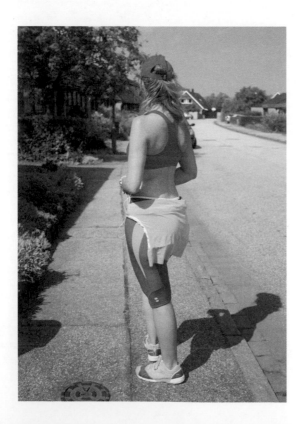

Stepping Out the Door

There are many more reasons to run than not to run, but those first tentative steps will be the toughest you will ever take. Stepping out on to the street in what feels like full view of all the neighbours is certainly not easy, but you'll soon discover that either no one is watching or, if they are, they are doing so with admiration!

Top Tip

If you feel really self-conscious about running, hit the streets early in the morning or after dark – just make sure you still follow basic safety rules.

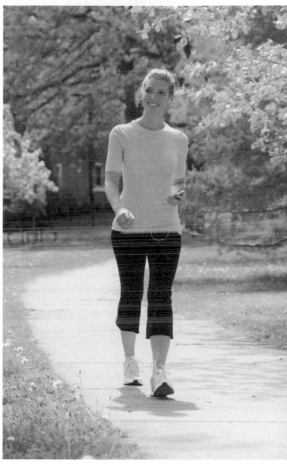

Run/Walk

Runners never walk, surely? Actually, they do. You may never see the likes of Usain Bolt strolling the last few metres of a race, but most mere mortals can quite legitimately drop their pace to a walk when they need to.

Start Slow

Depending on your base level of fitness, your running adventures may begin with what can only be described as a walk. There is nothing wrong with that, but do try to get into the habit of thinking of this as 'your *run*'. After a couple of days of walking your chosen route, pick up the pace just for a short

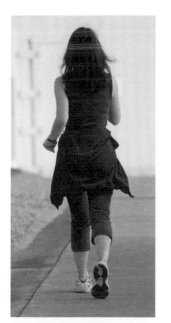

section – maybe no more than a minute or two at first. In no time at all, you will find yourself running the entire route.

Breaking the Pace

Even once you consider yourself a fully fledged runner, there are times when slowing to a walk can be beneficial. Mild cramps or a stitch can usually be 'walked out' in just a few minutes; running through them can make matters worse and might end your run completely. Never be afraid of taking a walking break. If your legs feel like they simply won't run another step, reduce your speed.

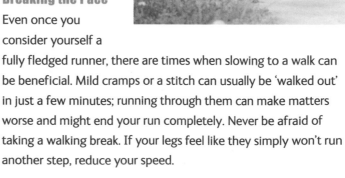

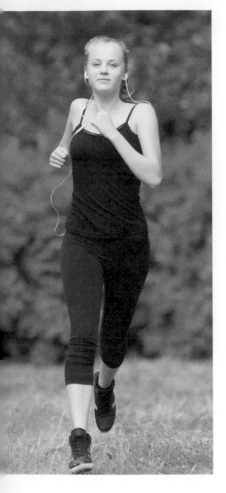

Morning or Evening?

One of the great joys of running is that it can fit in easily around your daily routine. By nature, most of us fall into one of two categories: early bird or night owl. Which you are will probably influence when you run. Both ends of the day have their merits: a dawn run brings a sense of freedom and the joy of seeing a new day emerging around you; an evening run can do wonders for unwinding mentally after a tough day at work. During the summer months, running in either the morning or evening will help avoid the heat.

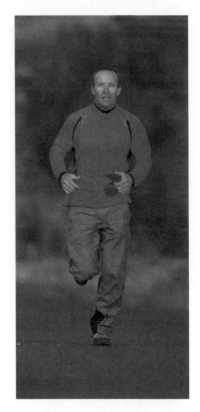

Safety

Safety should be your number-one priority on every run. Running safety is mostly common sense, but even a momentary lapse can spell disaster and taking some simple steps will ensure a safe and happy run.

 MP3 players: Only ever listen to music on a run when you are *certain* it is safe to do so, and never when running in the road.

 Run against the traffic: If you are running in the road, you are vulnerable. Always run on the side of the road where you are facing oncoming traffic.

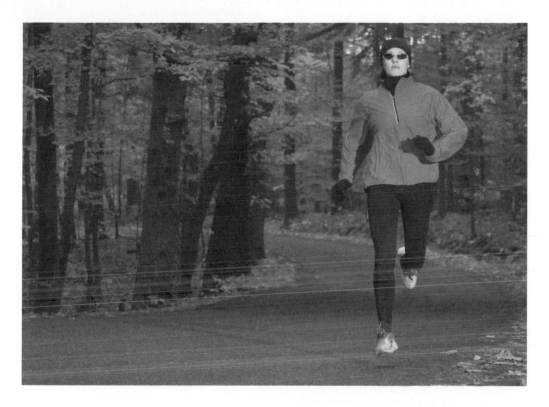

☑ **Be seen**: Running at night and in poor visibility means wearing 3, high-visibility clothing and even small clip-on lights. Make yourself as visible as possible.

☑ **Stay in contact**: When exploring more isolated routes, take a mobile phone. Public phone boxes aren't as common as they used to be.

☑ **Beware driveways**: When running on pavements, stay alert for cars reversing from drives.

☑ **Take a running mate**: If you are concerned about isolated routes, always run with someone else.

Be Inspired

'Practise yourself in little things, and thence proceed to greater.'
Epictetus, philosopher

Make your route known: It is always best to let someone know roughly where you are intending to go and how long you are likely to be.

Make a noise: A small attack alarm or whistle can be a sensible precaution.

Pay attention: It is all too easy to allow a car to pass, only to step out in front of a second vehicle. Stay alert.

Carry identification: This is vital in case of an emergency – consider something as simple as writing your phone number inside a shoe; paramedics will know to check.

ICE: If you carry a mobile phone, enter a contact as ICE (In Case of Emergency) with a relevant contact number – again, paramedics know to check for this.

Rights of way: Always check on a map for rights of way, as online satellite maps can be (literally) misleading.

Silent cyclists: Cyclists make little noise, but an impact with one can be as devastating as with a car. Stay alert on likely cycle routes.

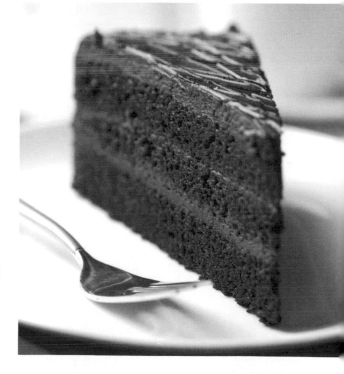

Food

Good nutrition goes hand in hand with good hydration for a runner. Food and drink fuel a run and their importance should never be underestimated. Taking up running does not necessarily mean radical changes to all other areas of your daily life, but, as your health consciousness grows, you'll become increasingly aware of your body's needs and to get the most out of your training certain changes to your diet are inevitable.

A Runner's Diet

Nutrition really means two things to a runner: the food eaten specifically before (or during) a run, and daily healthy eating. Sensible eating – particularly if you are running to lose weight – should become second nature to a runner, so it is useful to understand just a little of the science behind food.

Ditching the Junk

An important part of a healthy lifestyle involves cutting down on foods that are high in saturated fats, sugars and other 'junk' components. The occasional treat – a calorific Indian takeaway or chocolate cake – is not a problem, and can be a motivating reward, but it's important to be aware of what you're putting into your body.

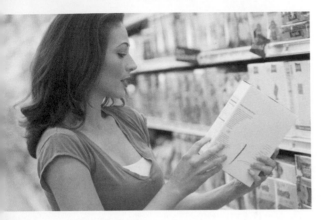

Building the Carbohydrates

Carbohydrates (or simply 'carbs') are one of the primary classes of nutrient, and a vital fuel for running. They are converted into glucose, which supplies energy to organs, tissues and muscles.

Simple and Complex Carbohydrates

Carbohydrates are divided into simple and complex types. Simple carbs are quick-release energy sources, and do not usually supply any other nutrients or fibre. They are generally found in sugars, which go by many names, including lactose, fructose and sucrose. Complex carbs (or starches) are absorbed and released into the body at a slower, more even rate and should form the basis for a good running diet.

Sources of Complex Carbohydrates

- ☑ Wholemeal pasta
- ☑ Wholemeal bread
- ☑ Potatoes
- ☑ Vegetables
- ☑ Cereals
- ☑ Rice

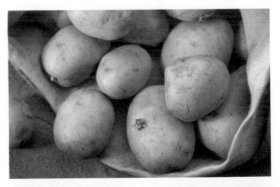

Top Tip

Beware of hidden fats, sugar and salt – many processed foods contain all three in sometimes alarming quantities. Runners read labels!

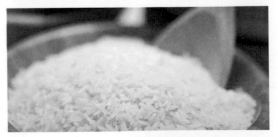

Watching the Protein

Although protein is vital for building and repairing muscles, a runner's diet requires less protein than a non-runner's. The food we eat today really contains too much protein and, as the majority of your running energy comes from complex carbohydrates, excess protein will be turned to fat and can lead to kidney problems and dehydration.

Protein is still important in helping carbohydrates to metabolize (and therefore become useful to the body), but only in a ratio of around four parts carbohydrates to one part protein. This 4:1 ratio is most commonly found in sports-nutrition products such as running bars.

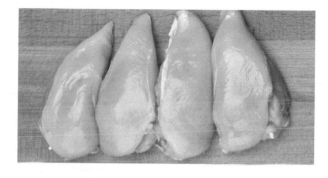

Sources of Protein

- Milk
- Meat
- Fish
- Eggs
- Nuts
- Vegetables

Top Tip

Low-carb diets (or no-carb diets, such as Atkins) are completely incompatible with running. Never combine the two!

Finding the Balance

A runner's diet will generally comprise a greater percentage of carbohydrates than an average diet (around 65 per cent compared to just 50 per cent), combined with less protein (15 per cent instead of 20 per cent) and less fat (20 per cent rather than approximately 30 per cent for non-runners). However, try not to get too preoccupied with crunching the numbers – just stay aware of the balance in your diet.

Vegetarian Runners

Generally, vegetarians pay greater attention to their diet and are more aware of their body's requirements. However, there are a few areas of potential deficiency that should be watched:

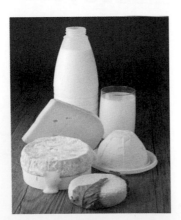

 Amino acids: These help maintain performance and aid in repairing the body, as well as boosting immunity. Meat eaters get their amino acids from protein-rich meats and fish, but vegetarians can rely on dairy, tofu products and baked potatoes.

 Iron: Vegetable, fruit and cereals rich in iron can be better absorbed by the body in conjunction with vitamin C. Supplements for vegetarians can be useful for striking the balance.

 Vitamin B12: Essential for both muscle repair and oxygen delivery, B12 is not found in plant foods, but dairy products should provide sufficient amounts – otherwise, consider vitamin supplements.

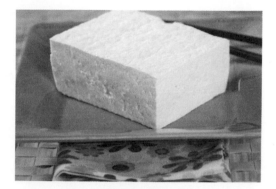

✔ **Zinc:** Along with iron, zinc is one of the most crucial minerals in our diet, and some studies have suggested that vegetarians may lack suitable levels. Look to tofu, wheat germ and wholegrain foods to boost levels.

✔ **Protein:** Wholegrain and soy products, along with beans, legumes (lentils, etc.) and nuts, are useful sources of protein without recourse to meat.

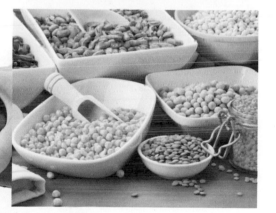

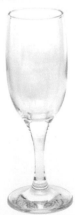

Eating for an Event

You should pay particular attention to your diet in the lead-up to an organized event – whether it is your first 5k or your tenth marathon. The week before a race is considered to be the 'fuelling stage', and whilst there is a great deal of misinformation and hype surrounding this, a few simple rules do apply:

✔ **Avoid all alcohol in the week prior to a race.**
✔ **Concentrate on a 4:1 ratio of complex carbohydrates to proteins.**

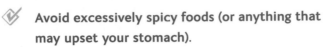
- ✔ Avoid excessively spicy foods (or anything that may upset your stomach).
- ✔ Watch your caffeine intake to avoid dehydration.
- ✔ Eat fruit, but avoid too much of it, as it can cause digestive problems.

Be Inspired

'If you can dream it, you can do it.'
*Walt Disney,
filmmaker*

Carb-loading

When you take up running, you'll pretty quickly come across the term 'carb-loading'. This refers to stocking up on complex carbohydrates such as pasta, rice and potatoes in the days before a big run. It might come as some surprise, then, that it didn't make the dietary list above.

Only a finite amount of energy (glycogen) from dietary carbohydrates can be stored in the muscles and liver – enough to fuel somewhere between 60 and 90 minutes of exercise. So, although it is a good idea to keep this topped up with pasta, etc. before an event, there is no way of storing additional amounts for use on the big day. A little overeating before a long run won't hurt, but there is no magic fuelling to be had from carb-loading.

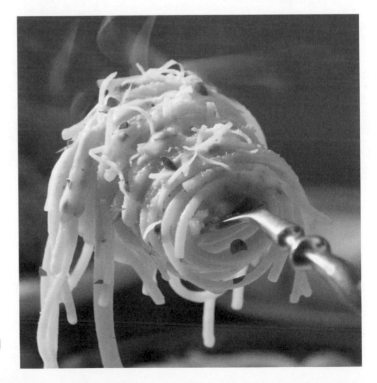

Eating on the Run

Because of the body's limited store of energy, which differs from person to person, replenishing your spent fuel by consuming sports-specific gels or bars is an important part of the runner's routine. Once the preserve of elite athletes, the consumer market for these products has exploded in the last decade.

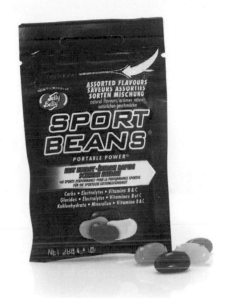

Sugar Rush

Sports beans – similar to traditional sweet jelly beans – are available in a variety of flavours, as are semi-solid gels that can be chewed like a cube of jelly. Both work in near-identical ways to gels. Some runners swear by nothing fancier than old-fashioned jelly babies, but don't be tempted by sweets rather than sports formulated products, as they are likely to deliver short, sharp spikes of sugar energy that is rapidly burned by the body.

Running Gels

Running or sports gels come in many varieties, but they are all designed to provide a fast delivery of energy during a run. The exact combination of ingredients varies from manufacturer to manufacturer, but will typically contain:

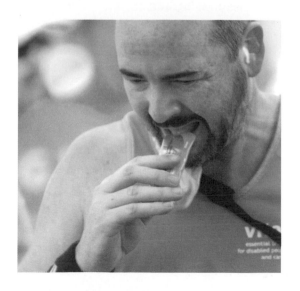

Be Inspired

'It's always too early to quit.'
Dr Norman Vincent Peale,
author

- ☑ Water
- ☑ A source of energy from sugar (such as maltodextrin)
- ☑ Natural flavouring
- ☑ Gelling agents (such as xanthan gum)
- ☑ Acidity regulators
- ☑ Preservatives
- ☑ Sweetener
- ☑ Sodium chloride (salt)
- ☑ Antioxidant
- ☑ Colourings

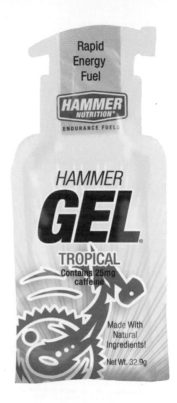

A typical 60-ml sachet of gel will deliver around 22 g of carbohydrates and be in the region of 90–100 calories. When choosing your gel, consider the following:

- ☑ **Natural ingredients**: Avoid artificial ingredients whenever possible.

- ☑ **Thickness (viscosity)**: Some gels are almost too thick to swallow!

- ☑ **Taste**: Very few gels taste good, so aim for at least 'okay' on the flavour scale.

- ☑ **Size**: Larger, weightier gels may be more watery (and easier to swallow), but thicker gels are lighter and smaller to carry.

- ☑ **Price**: Most gels cost between £1 and £1.50; buy in bulk to save money.

Top Tip

Never test a new gel on a race or long run; neither are the right time to discover you hate your latest purchase.

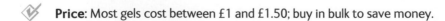

Energy Bars

Energy bars provide an excellent alternative to gels (which many find unpalatable) and generally contain a percentage of protein, which works in conjunction with the carbohydrates to speed up energy delivery. On the downside, energy bars are bulkier and heavier to carry.

To an even greater extent than gels, the ingredients in energy bars vary enormously, so you are far more likely to find a bar than a gel to match your mood and taste. When choosing an energy bar, consider the following:

- **Natural ingredients:** Many offer organic credentials, so the healthier, the better.

- **Taste:** If it does not taste good, it will not get eaten and will not help your run.

- **Texture:** How does a bar's texture change in extremes of temperature?

- **Size:** Check to see how much energy you are getting for the weight.

- **Allergies:** Many bars contain nuts, so check the packaging for allergy advice.

- **Price:** Most bars cost between £1.50 and £2.50, so buy in bulk to save money.

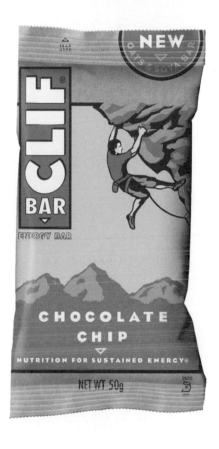

Top Tip

Do not confuse recovery bars with running bars – although similar, they contain different ratios of ingredients (mostly carbohydrates and proteins) and are designed for different purposes.

Hydration

Water accounts for about 60 per cent of body weight in adult males and 50–55 per cent in females. Lean muscles and the brain are around 75 per cent water, blood is 81 per cent and even bones are 22 per cent. Water fuels every part of the body and, without sufficient water, things can quickly go wrong.

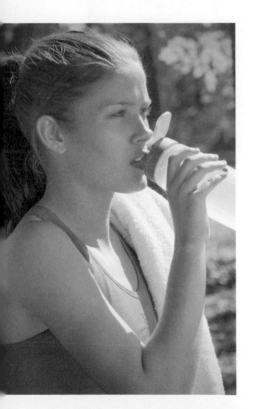

The Importance of Water

It is almost impossible to overstate the importance of good hydration to a runner, so taking a few minutes to understand a little of the science behind this is highly recommended.

What Does Water Do?

Water serves several key functions in the body.

- ✔ Helps weight loss; preventing confusion between hunger and thirst.
- ✔ Flushes toxins from the body.
- ✔ Moisturizes the skin and helps maintain elasticity.
- ✔ Helps maintain cushioning and lubrication in the joints.
- ✔ Reduces the risk of kidney and bladder infections.
- ✔ Improves circulation.
- ✔ Regulates body temperature.

Why We Sweat

Unlike other animals, which roll around in mud (pigs) or flap their ears (elephants), humans regulate their body temperature via the sweat mechanism. In hot conditions or during exercise, sweat glands – some 2.6 million in the average adult – produce a fluid that is transported to the surface of the skin, where it evaporates and cools us down.

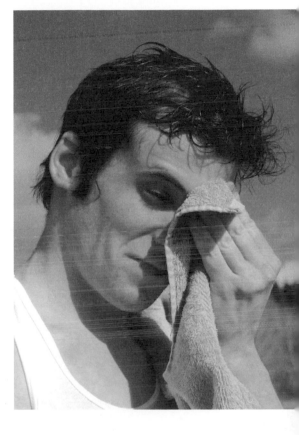

How Much Do You Sweat?

The amount of sweat produced varies between individuals, and is also dependent on both the duration of exercise and weather conditions.

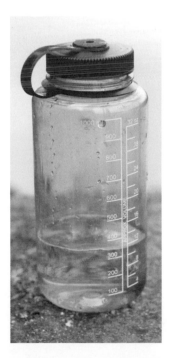

However, as a rough guide, during a moderately fast run on a warm day, a person will sweat in the region of 500–600 ml per hour.

The amount we sweat is directly proportional to the amount of water that should be replaced, so it can be useful to more accurately calculate a 'sweat rate'. Do so as follows:

 Weigh yourself naked in kilograms.

 Make a note of exactly how much water you have in your bottle in millilitres.

 Run at the pace for which you want to calculate your sweat rate for one hour.

- ✅ Make a note of how much water you have consumed (in millilitres).
- ✅ Wipe excess sweat from your skin and weigh yourself again.
- ✅ Sweat loss (in millilitres) = body weight before exercise (in kilograms) – body weight after exercise (kilograms) + water consumed during exercise.

Top Tip

For really accurate sweat rates, repeat the sweat test a few times and take an average. It can be useful to know your sweat rate for various weather (temperature) conditions.

Before a Run

Make sure that you are adequately hydrated before any form of exercise – pay particular attention if you are running first thing in the morning, as your body slowly dehydrates overnight. Avoid coffee and alcohol, as both contribute to dehydration, but, equally, avoid excessive water, as this will 'slosh' uncomfortably on the run and can lead to frequent toilet breaks.

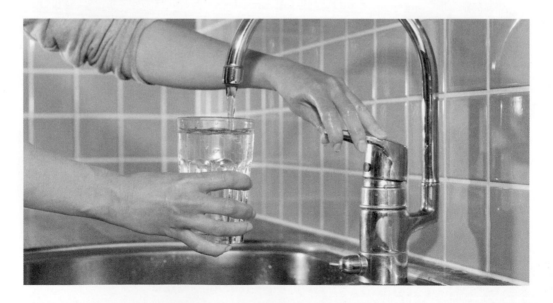

On the Run

Making a note of your sweat rate, ensure that you are replacing enough fluids on an hourly basis. Drink little and often – sipping regularly from a bottle will encourage the habit of good hydration. If you wait until you feel thirsty, you've left it too long.

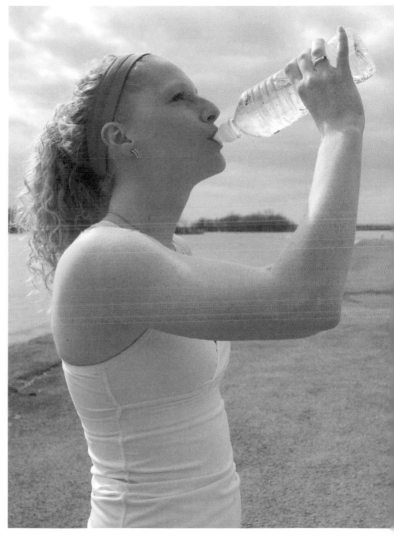

Post-run

Avoid the temptation to gulp down water after a run, and in particular avoid ice-cold water, as this may cause stomach cramps. Continue to drink regularly through the day and, again, avoid coffee and alcohol.

Salting it Out

Although plain water goes a long way to rehydrating the body, a great deal of salt (a combination that includes sodium, potassium and magnesium rather than the 'table' variety) is lost during exercise. It is important, especially on long runs, to replace these as quickly as possible. Most sports drinks include these body salts, but it is also worth using salt-replacement tablets, which can be dissolved in a regular water bottle.

Sports Drinks

Although basic sports and running drinks have been around for half a century, the market has grown beyond all recognition in the last 10 years, despite the fact that they remain a fairly simple mix of carbohydrates (energy from sugars), electrolytes (body salts), water and flavourings.

Which Tonic?

Whatever else a sport drink may offer (an added caffeine kick, for example), there are three basic types:

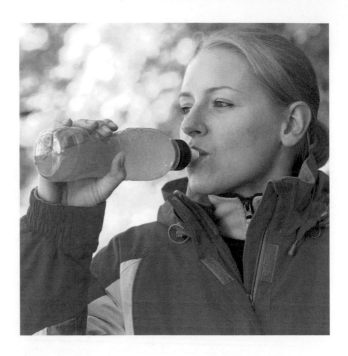

☑ **Hypotonic drinks**: These can be absorbed much more quickly than plain water because their ratio of carbohydrates and electrolytes is *less* than the body's. They do not offer the same energy surge as isotonic or hypertonic drinks, but they do replace fluids quickly and are best suited for use during low-intensity and hot runs.

☑ **Isotonic drinks**: These contain a balance of carbohydrates and electrolytes near-identical to that of the body. They are absorbed at about the same rate as water, but have the advantage of containing sugar-based energy. They work best for higher-intensity workouts, strenuous runs or races, and deliver a greater energy boost.

☑ **Hypertonic drinks**: These are best suited to post-exercise recovery, as they are absorbed relatively slowly but help to replenish energy and replace salts lost through sweating.

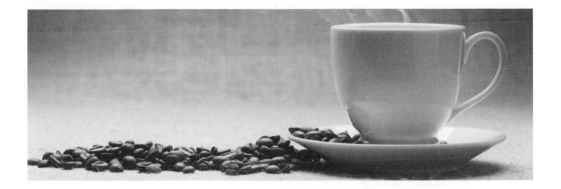

Is Caffeine Good for Runners?

Some sports drinks and virtually all 'energy' drinks contain caffeine – usually about the same amount found in a single shot of espresso. There is some evidence to suggest that small doses bring benefits such as increased VO2Max (the body's ability to absorb oxygen) and even lactic threshold (the point at which your muscles tire), but these are short-lived. Caffeine also produces a rush of energy, but this too is short-lived, and too much caffeine can cause a range of less desirable results, including raised blood pressure and upset stomachs.

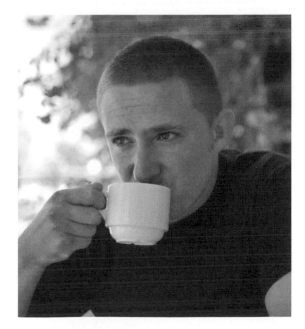

Top Tip
Avoid more than a single cup of coffee before a run, as it can contribute to dehydration. Be aware that tea, even some herbal teas, contains a percentage of caffeine.

How to Structure a Run

Depending on a range of factors (including your motivation for running), the structure of a run can take many forms. Interval or hill reps have their own combinations of drills, whilst a good trail run will largely be determined by the changing terrain. However, the structure of almost any run can be defined by five sections: pre-run warm-up or stretch, running warm-up, the run, running cool-down, post-run cool-down and stretch.

Pre-run Warm-up and Stretching

The usefulness of stretching before you run is a matter of some debate. Overzealous stretching of cold muscles can cause injury, and in most cases the warm-up stage can be more efficiently incorporated into the opening 10 minutes or so of the run itself.

Light stretching might be beneficial before a short, sharp run – a sprint or a 5k race at which you are aiming for a record time – but most real benefit from a pre-run warm-up is psychological. Spending five minutes 'getting into the zone' can ease the transition from a busy day of work to a stress-busting evening run.

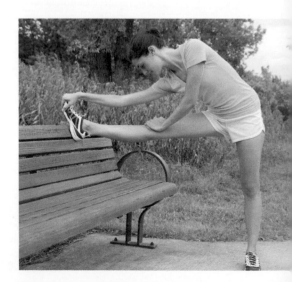

Be Inspired
'Either you run the day
or the day runs you.'
Jim Rohn, entrepreneur

Running Warm-up

Unless you are taking part in a race, it's vital to spend time finding your pace to warm up tight muscles at the start of your run. However mentally prepared you might feel, there is always an element of 'shock to the system' that can be eased by starting slowly. A more languid start will begin raising your heart rate and temperature as your blood flow increases for more effective delivery of oxygen to the active muscles. Five to 10 minutes of gentle running should be enough.

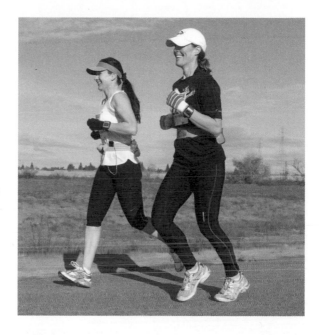

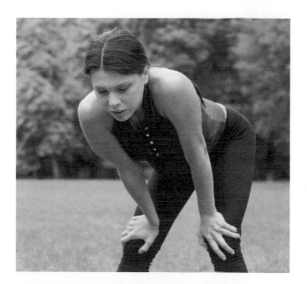

Running Cool-down

A sprint finish on any route (even just back to your door) is a huge temptation – and one that is best avoided. It is all too easy to injure yourself in the final few moments of a run that has otherwise gone to plan; slowing down in the final five to 10 minutes will allow your heart rate, temperature and breathing to gradually return to normal. Walking out the last few minutes will begin the recovery process.

Post-run Stretching

Stretching after a run is crucial for avoiding injury. This simple 10-minute routine should form the basis of every post-run stretch. Be sure to keep things relaxed, and never stretch or hold a stretch if you feel any pain or discomfort beyond a mild tension.

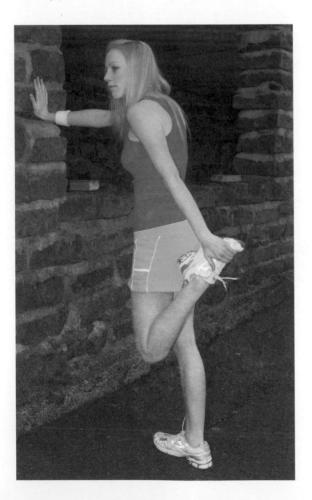

Quadriceps (Thigh)

- ✔ **Stand facing a wall with feet close together**.
- ✔ **Support yourself with left hand against the wall**.
- ✔ **Bend your right leg up backwards**.
- ✔ **Grasp your ankle with your right hand and pull your heel close to your bottom**.
- ✔ **Hold gently in position and slightly bend both knees**.
- ✔ **Hold for 20 seconds**.
- ✔ **Release and repeat for left leg**.
- ✔ **Repeat three times for each leg**.

Top Tip

Feeling self-conscious about the slow run or walk back to your house? Plenty of watch-checking or GPS button-pushing will keep you busy and make you feel like a 'real' runner again.

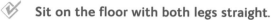

Outer Calf

- Sit on the floor with both legs straight.
- Loop a large towel (or elasticated exercise band) around the ball of one foot.
- Gently pull the towel towards you, flexing the foot back with the toes pointing towards the knee.
- Hold for 20 seconds.
- Release and repeat for other foot.
- Repeat three times for each foot.

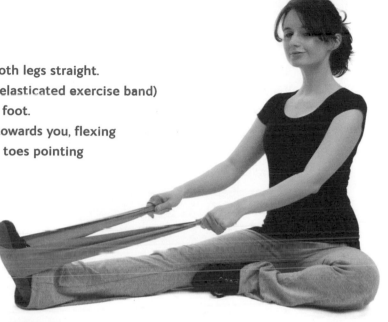

Inner Calf

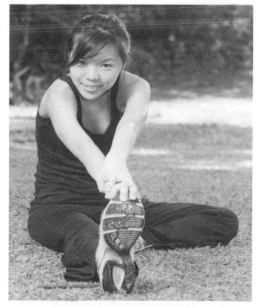

- Sit on the floor with left leg straight and the right bent at around 45 degrees, so that the right heel is almost in line with the left knee.
- Gently stretch forward and grasp the ball of the right foot.
- Keeping the right heel on the floor, gently pull the foot towards you.
- Hold for 20 seconds.
- Release and repeat for left foot.
- Repeat three times on each side.

Achilles Tendon

- Sit on the floor with your left leg straight.
- Bend the right leg so that the foot slides as close as possible to your bottom.
- Keep the right heel against the floor.
- Gently grasp your right foot and pull towards your body.
- Hold for 20 seconds.
- Release and repeat for left side.
- Repeat three times on each side.

Hamstring

- Lie flat on your back.
- Bend the right knee to around 45 degrees, keeping the foot flat on the floor.
- Keeping your hips flat against the floor, lift your left leg straight up in the air.
- Hold gently with both hands around the back of the knee or thigh.
- Gently point the toes towards the ceiling.
- Pull your left leg gently towards you, holding for 20 seconds.
- Release and repeat for the right leg.
- Repeat three times on each side.

Top Tip

If time is short, observe the bare minimum – five minutes slow-pace run to start, three to five minutes slow-pace run to end, five to 10 minutes of post-run stretching.

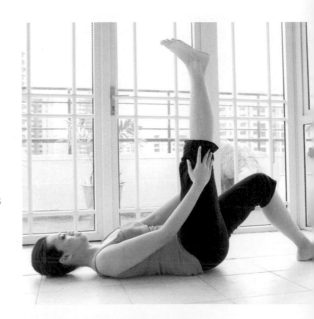

Cross Training

Many types of exercise can help improve your running – building general fitness, stamina and muscles, and aiding mental preparation too. A sensible 'whole-body' approach to running and training will see quicker results and make running easier and more enjoyable. A well-structured training programme should always include cross training, as this provides a break in routine and, as it generally involves less impact than running, it can drastically help to reduce the chances of injury.

Cycling

Cycling is an excellent way of increasing your stamina and all-round fitness. It is low impact, which can help in avoiding many of the most common running injuries, and will build many of the muscle groups needed for running. However, be careful not to overdo cycling, as it can 'unbalance' the combination of leg muscles used for running.

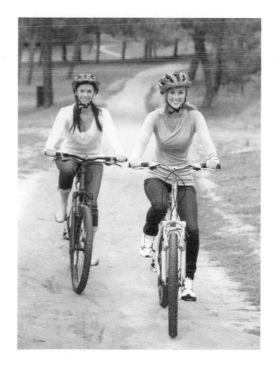

Benefits of Cycling

- ☑ **Improves lung and heart functions**
- ☑ **Builds leg and core muscles**
- ☑ **Low impact**
- ☑ **Great for route-planning your runs**

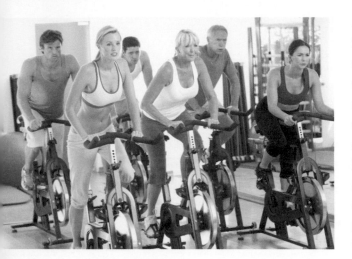

Spinning

Spinning is an organized group exercise class based on fixed-wheel bikes, usually accompanied by music. Just as with cycling, it helps build all-round fitness and is relatively low impact, but as it is a group activity it has the advantage of being both social and highly motivational. Most spinning sessions combine a mix of fast cycling and slow hill climbs, providing similar benefits to interval training (*see* page 40).

Benefits of Spinning

 Fun and motivational
 Improves lung and heart functions
 Builds leg and core muscles
 Low impact
 Works as interval training

Swimming

Because swimming is impact free (the water supports the body's weight), injured runners can use it to maintain fitness to a very high level. For general training, it builds stamina quickly and can help improve breathing techniques. Although unlikely to build leg strength, swimming does build core (stomach), shoulder and upper-back

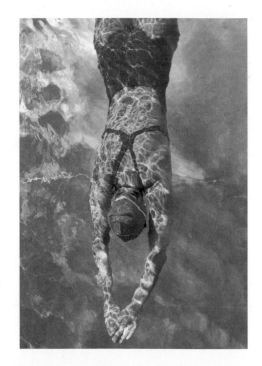

muscles – all of which perform a function in running. Swimming can also be a fun and relaxing way to spend time on a day that otherwise might not count as training.

Benefits of Swimming

 Impact free
 Builds back and core muscles
 Maintains fitness during injury
 Improves lung and heart functions

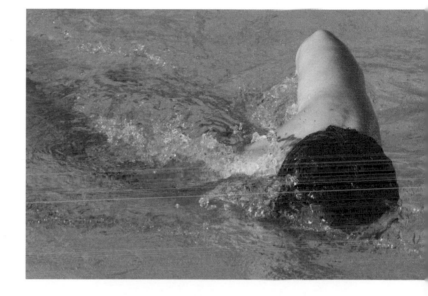

Aqua-jogging

Aqua-jogging – literally running in a pool – brings many advantages to both training and, if it is your goal, weight loss. Many local pools run special sessions, so there is no danger of getting in the way of swimmers and less likelihood of feeling self-conscious. Because the exercise is virtually impact free, it is one of the best ways of maintaining fitness during injury, and because water offers six times the resistance of air, evidence suggests that almost double the number of calories are burned per hour compared to running.

Benefits of Aqua-jogging

 Impact free
 Perfect for recovery
 Maintains fitness during injury
 Builds leg muscles

Be Inspired

'Even if you fall on your face, you're still moving forward.'
Victor Kiam, entrepreneur

Treadmill

There are runners who love them and runners who hate them, but, used wisely, a treadmill has much in its favour. When the weather is bad, there can be no excuse not to put in a few miles on a treadmill, and they are also an ideal place to try out new kit such as shoes.

Benefits of the Treadmill

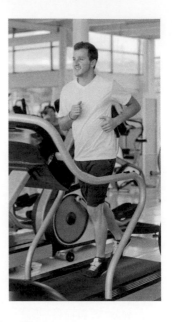

 Easily controlled, steady pace
 Year-round and weatherproof
✓ **Quickly builds strength and speed**

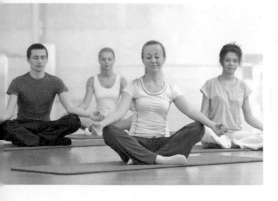

Yoga

Part of the 'whole-body' approach to running, yoga also helps with mental preparation and a general sense of wellbeing. In addition to being relaxing, yoga can help build the core muscles around the stomach, sides and lower back, which are the foundations for a strong body and vital to good running. Yoga teaches excellent breathing techniques that can be useful in training. It also improves concentration, circulation and flexibility.

Benefits of Yoga

 Relaxing
 Improves core muscles and circulation
 Builds good breathing techniques
 Helps flexibility to avoid injury

Top Tip

Combine as many types of cross training as possible for maximum benefit and to keep things interesting.

Putting Your Running Into Action

Now it's time to put your running into action. Following the simple plans below will kick-start your routine based on three common goals: running for general health and for weight loss, to improve stamina (distance or time running) and to increase speed.

General Health and Weight-Loss Plan

Weight loss is achieved only through a combination of exercise and diet – put very simply, 'eat less, move more'. Running to lose weight is incredibly motivating; although the results will not be instant, you can record your progress and follow through on targets. This is also an excellent plan if your motivation is simple all-round health and fitness, in which case you may also add some extra cross training or a gentle, short-run day.

The Goal

In addition to the obvious weight loss, the goal with this eight-week plan is to bring your maximum run length up to a comfortable 30 minutes – a great base time from which to grow your running (and shrink your waist).

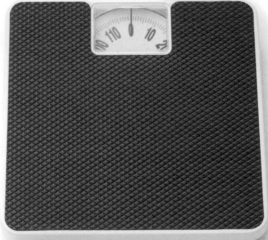

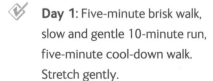

The Plan

✅ **Day 1**: Five-minute brisk walk, slow and gentle 10-minute run, five-minute cool-down walk. Stretch gently.

✅ **Day 2**: Rest.

✅ **Day 3**: Five-minute brisk walk, slow and gentle 10-minute run, five-minute cool-down walk. Stretch gently.

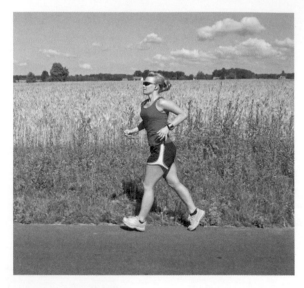

✅ **Day 4**: Rest.

✅ **Day 5**: Cross train with 30-minute swim, 30–45-minute cycle or 45–60-minute walk.

✅ **Day 6**: Five-minute brisk walk, slow and gentle 10-minute run, five-minute cool-down walk. Stretch gently.

✅ **Day 7**: Rest.

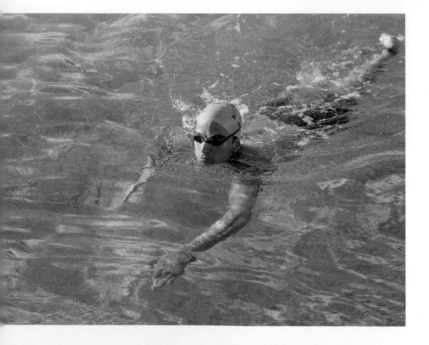

Week 2: Keeping day one the same, increase the run section of days three and six from 10 to 12 minutes. The brisk walk warm-up and cool-down may be stepped up to a very slow run.

Week 3: Keeping day one the same to start the running week gently, increase the length of run on days three and six by around two minutes, to bring the total run time up to 14 minutes. Another cross-training day can be introduced on day seven – try to keep things varied and interesting.

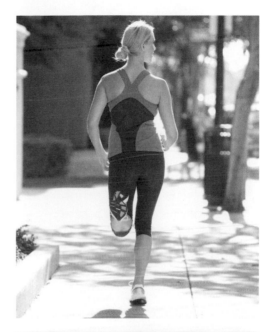

Week 4: Increase the day-one run to the time of the previous week's days three and six (around 14 minutes). Increase your run time on day three to 16 minutes and day five to 18 minutes. Including the warm-up and cool-down walk, you should now be out for around 33 minutes!

Week 5: Time to step things up by increasing all three runs by 10 per cent – day one 15–16 minutes, day three 18 minutes and day six 20 minutes. Try to increase the length of your cross training too, but don't overdo things.

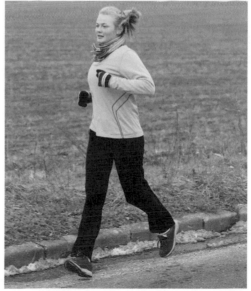

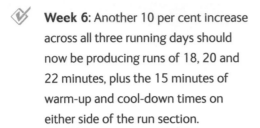
Week 6: Another 10 per cent increase across all three running days should now be producing runs of 18, 20 and 22 minutes, plus the 15 minutes of warm-up and cool-down times on either side of the run section.

Week 7: Keeping days one and three at around the same duration (18–20 minutes), try stepping up the day-six time to 25 minutes; keep your pace as slow as necessary and just aim for your time goal.

Week 8: Time to hit your target. Again keeping the first two runs at around the 20-minute mark, push your day-six run all the way through to the full 30 minutes.

Top Tip

Continue to increase running time beyond this plan if you wish, but keep at least one run short and increase amounts of either time or distance only by around 10–15 per cent a week.

Keys to Success

- Keep things casual and relaxed.
- Do not panic, but do focus on your goals.
- Cross training helps to break things up and adds variety.
- Rule of thumb: one mile burns approximately 100 calories.
- Maintain a sensible approach to diet.
- Keep a diary – log your runs, thoughts and weight.
- Share the joy – tell friends 'I'm a runner!'
- Do not expect instant results.
- Keep hydrated.

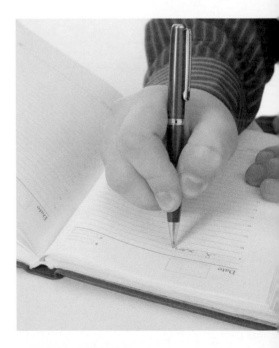

Stamina Plan

This plan assumes that you are already capable of running at a steady pace for 45 minutes. If you are not yet at this stage, follow the weight loss/health plan until you reach this level. Improving your stamina to run further or for longer is all about making small but frequent

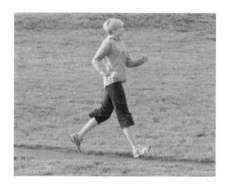

increases in your performance. Take things slowly and concentrate on the amount of time you are running for – improving your speed over distance can wait.

The Goal

This plan follows *slow* increases to move your overall running time up from 45 to 90 minutes. To take things further, follow the pattern, but make increases on your longest run by around 10–15 per cent a week.

The Plan

 Day 1: Run slowly to warm up for five to 10 minutes. On a hill with a gentle to moderate incline, run for three minutes uphill, two minutes down and repeat twice, making a total of 15 minutes. Ten-minute cool-down run and stretch.

 Day 2: Rest.

 Day 3: This will always be your longest run of the week. Run slowly to warm up for five to 10 minutes. Pick up the pace to moderate (you should still be able to comfortably hold a conversation) and run for 45 minutes. Ten-minute slow cool-down run and stretch.

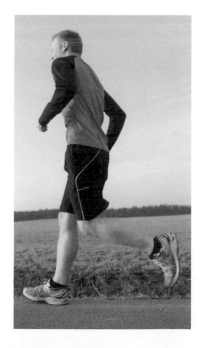

Day 4: Rest.

Day 5: A shorter 'recovery' run – five minutes warm-up, 30 minutes at a slow, easy pace, ten-minute cool-down run and stretch.

Day 6: Aim for an hour of low-intensity cross training: a bike ride is ideal.

Day 7: Rest.

Week 2: As for week one, but increase your long run on day three from 45 to 50 minutes.

Week 3: Repeat again, raising the long run by a further five minutes to 55 minutes. Take things slowly and remember to maintain warm-ups and cool-downs.

Week 4: To mix things up, switch the hill reps for gentle interval training: warm up for five to 10 minutes, run at a faster pace than on your long run (day three) for five minutes, slow the pace for three minutes and repeat twice more for a total time of 24 minutes. Cool-down stretch. Increase your long run on day three to 61 minutes (you have broken the one hour mark!) Increase the recovery run on day five to 35 minutes.

Week 5: Switch back to hill reps on day one, and increase your long run on day three to 67 minutes.

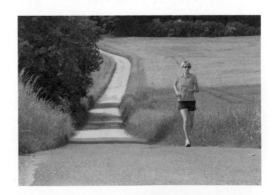

Week 6: Back to the intervals on day one (as in week four), increase the day-three long run to 74 minutes and the day-five slower recovery run to 40 minutes.

Week 7: Return to hill reps on day one, increase your long run (day three) to 82 minutes.

Week 8: Repeat week seven, but increase the day-three long run to 90 minutes and day-five slow recovery to 45 minutes.

Keys to Success

- Always warm up and cool down on each run.
- Do not forget to stretch.
- Keep a diary – log your runs and progress.
- Drink adequate water before, during *and* after exercise.
- Use energy gels and bars once you pass the 60-minute point.
- Rest days are vital for recovery.
- Do not be impatient – increasing stamina is a slow process.
- Only work on speed when you are comfortable with longer runs.

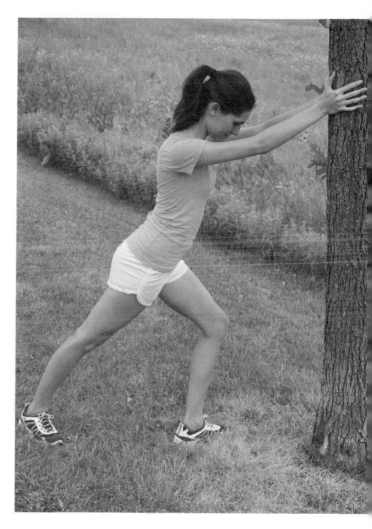

Top Tip

If you are a gym member, talk to staff about weight training or cross training for stamina. Be specific about your goals.

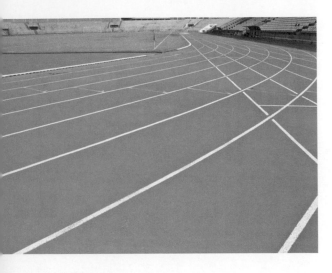

Speed Plan

This plan assumes that you are already capable of running at a steady pace for 35–45 minutes. If not, follow the weight loss/health plan until you have reached this level. Shifting up through the gears should not be daunting, and hitting that target speed is one of the most rewarding things a runner can do. Ideally, you will have access to a measured 400 m distance (such as a running track); if not, estimate the distance along an unbroken stretch of your usual running route.

The Goal

Use a combination of run types to slowly increase speed across eight weeks. If you are using this plan to train for a race, allow one full recovery week before the event.

The Plan

 Day 1: Run slowly to warm up for five to 10 minutes. Run your measured 400 m at a hard pace, followed by a second 400 m at a very slow run or walk (this is one 'interval'). Repeat the hard pace/slow run 400 m twice more for a total of three intervals. Ten-minute cool-down run and stretch.

 Day 2: Rest.

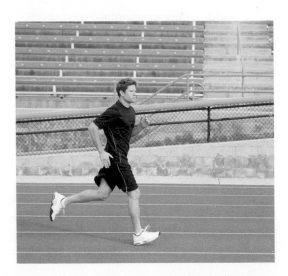

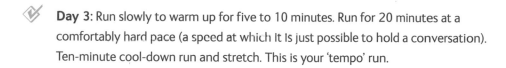

Day 3: Run slowly to warm up for five to 10 minutes. Run for 20 minutes at a comfortably hard pace (a speed at which it is just possible to hold a conversation). Ten-minute cool-down run and stretch. This is your 'tempo' run.

Day 4: Gentle cross training: a 30-minute swim or 45–60-minute bike ride will help improve heart and lungs.

Day 5: Rest.

Day 6: Run slowly to warm up for five to 10 minutes. Run at a gentle pace for 30 minutes and end with 10-minute slow cool-down run and stretch.

Day 7: Rest.

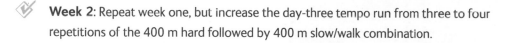

Week 2: Repeat week one, but increase the day-three tempo run from three to four repetitions of the 400 m hard followed by 400 m slow/walk combination.

Week 3: Repeat week two, increasing the 20-minute comfortably hard section of the tempo run to 22 minutes.

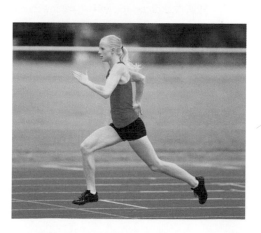

Week 4: Increase day-one intervals to five repetitions of 400 m hard/walk. Increase day-three tempo run by another two minutes to 24 minutes. Increase the gentle day-six run to 32 minutes.

Week 5: Continue with five repetitions of 400 m intervals on day one, increasing the tempo run by another two minutes. Switch to tougher cross training to increase heart rate – 30 minutes on the exercise bike, 20 minutes on the rowing machine or a 60-minute hard bike ride. Increase the day six gentle run to 34 minutes.

Week 6: Day one should now be six 400 m repetitions or hard/slow. Continue with the harder (heart rate-raising) cross-training and increase both the day-three (tempo) and day-six (gentle) runs by another two minutes.

Week 7: Repeat week six, again increasing both day-three (tempo) and day-six (gentle) runs by another two minutes.

Week 8: Repeat week seven, with a final increase of both day-three (tempo) and day-six (gentle) runs by another two minutes.

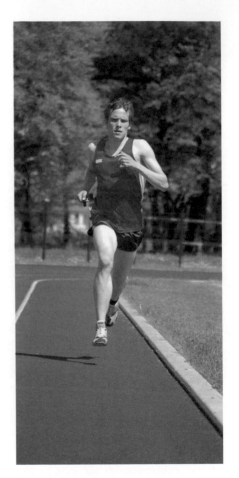

Keys to Success

- Always warm up and cool down on each run.
- Do not forget to stretch.
- Keep a diary – log your runs and progress.
- Drink adequate water before, during *and* after exercise.
- Rest days are vital for recovery.

Top Tip

If you are a member of a gym, talk to staff there about weight training for speed. Be specific about your goals.

Checklist

✔ **Check your fitness:** Take time to get some base measurements, such as blood pressure, weight and heart rate. This gives you a starting point against which to measure your progress.

✔ **Take the first steps:** Take things slowly – never be afraid to drop your pace and walk. Becoming a runner takes time and patience.

✔ **Safety:** Check that your route is safe and take all sensible precautions, especially when running at night.

✔ **Watch what you eat:** Pay careful attention to your diet, read food labels and listen to your body's needs.

✔ **Stay hydrated:** Check that you are drinking enough before, during and after running.

✔ **Identify your goals:** Look at your reasons for wanting to run. This makes it far easier to measure your progress.

✔ **Avoid injury:** Always warm up, cool down and stretch as part of your running routine.

✔ **Mix it up:** Cross training adds variety and helps to build all aspects of training. Make it fun.

Training & Advanced Running

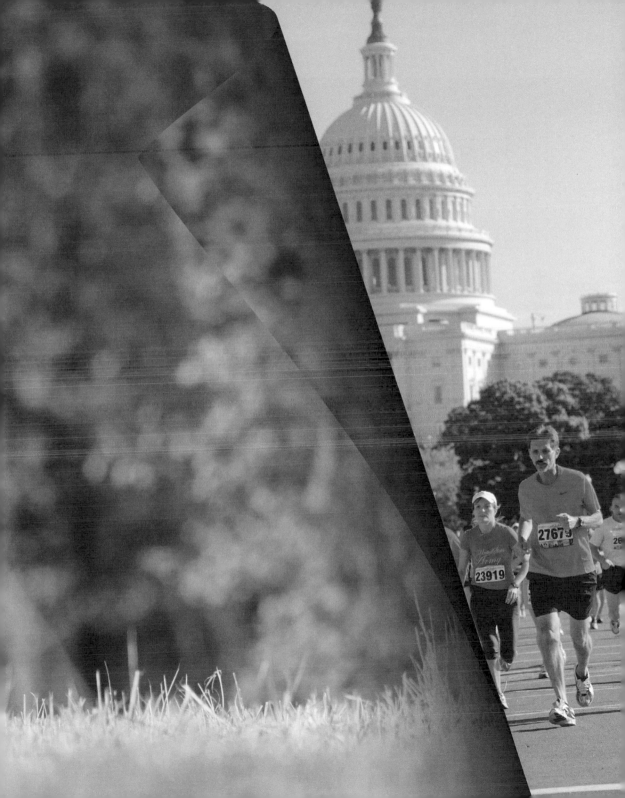

Moving on

Having achieved whatever goals you originally set – weight loss, fitness, time or distance – and 'become a runner', there will come a moment when you ask yourself what happens next. This is the time to evaluate what kind of runner you have become, and to set yourself some new goals.

What Kind of Runner Are You?

Runners can be divided into two quite distinct categories: sociable and loner. The kind of runner you have become is not necessarily determined by the kind of person you are in your day-to-day life – many 'party animals' find solace in the long, solo run, whilst those of a more reserved nature often find a more extrovert side to their personality in their running. You may surprise yourself when you stop and consider what type of runner you have become.

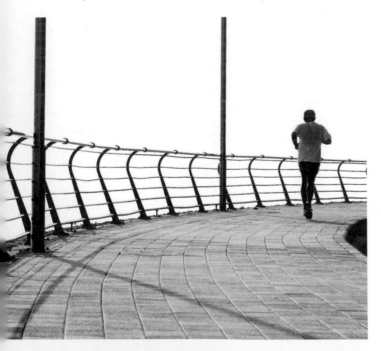

Be Inspired

'What you get by achieving your goals is not as important as what you become by achieving your goals.'
Henry David Thoreau, writer and philosopher

The Sociable Runner

Sharing your achievements and admiring those of others is truly motivating. The internet has brought together runners from around the world into a global community, allowing you to share your love of running with people you have never even met. Closer to home, a running club can provide added incentives, encouraging participation in a wide range of events and helping to push your running far beyond a point you may think possible.

Tips for the Sociable Runner

- **Hit the online forums**: Find your global running buddies.

- **Log your achievements online**: Compare your goals and beat your rivals.

- **Join a running club**: Enjoy the full social benefits of running.

- **Consider group exercise classes**: Spinning or circuit training are excellent.

- **Look for large events**: Sign up for event such as the Great North Run in Newcastle, England.

- **Start raising money**: Every step counts for charity.

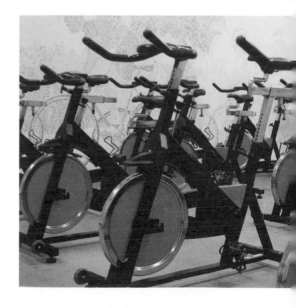

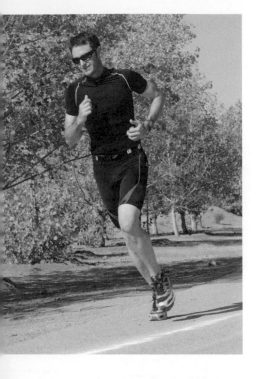

The Lone Runner

If you find yourself loving the solitude of an early evening run, with time alone to clear your head and rid yourself of the day's stress, then running clubs and large-scale events, with all their associated banner waving, are probably not for you. But even if you are your own best company on a run, do not shy away from learning from others; there are dozens of inspiring books on all levels of running (*see* page 252) and the internet is a great source of motivational blogs and forums, even if you choose not to actively participate.

Tips for the Lone Runner

- **Set your own goals and targets**: Compete only against yourself.

- **Log your runs online**: Keep your settings private.

- **Look for local runs**: For when you're feeling a little more sociable, these offer smaller groups and less 'fuss' than big clubs and events.

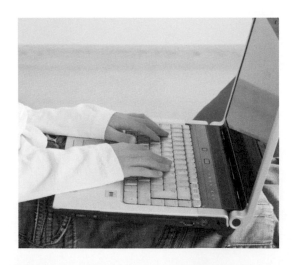

- **Consider cross training**: Keep it self-focused, such as cycling or swimming.

- **Explore ultra-marathons**: These may be perfect for you – the ultimate test of 'self'.

Extra Motivation

There are days when even the most dedicated runner may lack motivation. Keeping things fresh and interesting can be a challenge in itself, but a few simple steps will keep things moving. Two of the most motivational things to do are keeping a log or journal and joining a local club.

Runner's Log

Whether you are a sociable or lone runner, there is no better way of tracking your progress and chasing your goals than keeping a log of your running. At its simplest, this can be an old-fashioned diary in which you keep track of your times and miles covered, but far more flexible, motivating and accurate is joining one of the many online running communities. There is generally no cost involved in either registering for or using your online log (indeed, be wary of any that *do* charge), and with the increased use of both GPS watches and smartphone apps, you will even be able to update your status and distance automatically.

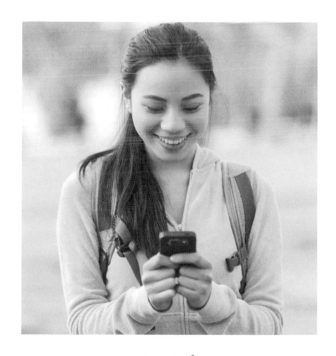

Top Tip
**Record the good and the bad.
Learn from your mistakes.**

Running Clubs

Joining a running club may seem like a daunting prospect, but almost without exception, clubs are friendly, welcoming and, above all, will give you that gentle push you need to take your running to the next level.

Advice and Information

Besides the obvious social benefits of meeting like-minded people, clubs are an invaluable source of advice and information on everything from shoes and kit to injury recovery and training.

Generally clubs meet a couple of times each week to undertake different types of run (perhaps a longer run one day and some faster speed training on another). There is never any obligation to do anything you don't feel comfortable with, nor any pressure to run at club events.

Try First

Clubs always offer free taster sessions and, if you do decide to take the plunge and join, fees are unlikely to be more than a few pounds a week. The relatively small annual fees can also be quickly recouped if you intend to enter races and events, as these invariably offer reduced 'affiliated runner rates' to club members.

Nutrition and Hydration

As your distances and the time you spend running increase, it is vital to maintain a diet that supports the level of exercise you are undertaking. Continue to monitor the balance of carbohydrates and protein in your diet, and always avoid junk foods when training hard for an event.

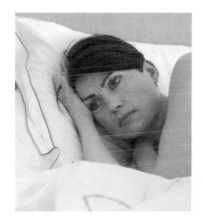

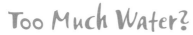

Salt for Sleep

It is not uncommon for runners who have suddenly increased the intensity of their training (perhaps in the lead-up to a race) to find that their sleep becomes disturbed. Some studies suggest this may be due to an imbalance of body salts – sodium, potassium, magnesium and zinc. Use rehydration salt tablets (available from high-street chemists) after long or hot runs to help rectify this.

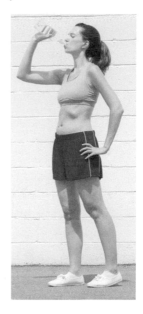

Too Much Water?

Although over-hydration is rare in day-to-day running, it is essential to understand that drinking excess water (anything much more than your sweat rate suggests – see page 155) can be extremely damaging to the body. In excess, plain water alone will dilute the body's salt combinations with potentially life-threatening consequences. Whilst dehydration is relatively easy to treat, over-hydration is not. Pay attention to your sweat rate and stick to your hydration plan.

Working the Core

There are many definitions for what exactly constitutes the core muscles, but broadly speaking they are the stomach, side and lower back muscles that form the foundation of strength throughout the body. Building the leg muscles with running (or additional cross training or weight training) is a great starting position, but a strong core is the foundation upon which long-term running is based.

Core Benefits

The key benefits to a strong core are:

 Encourages good posture
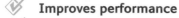 Improves performance
 Reduces back problems
Improves distance running

Weekly Routine

The simple set of four exercises outlined below should be included in your training plan at least once a week, particularly when working towards an endurance event such as a half-marathon or marathon. The clam exercise extends the workout through the glutes (bottom) – a much-neglected area.

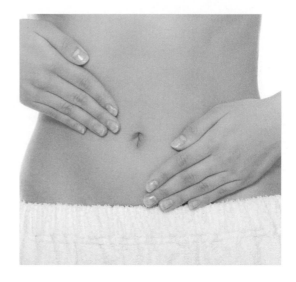

Top Tip
An extensive range of core exercises can be found online. Keep things varied and interesting.

Superman

- Lie face down on the floor with your arms straight out ahead.
- With your head facing forward, slowly lift your arms and legs up.
- Aim to hold both arms and legs straight, 20–25 cm (8–10 in) off the floor.
- Feel the stretch across the stomach muscles.
- Hold for 10 seconds
- Relax and remember to breathe.
- Repeat for a total of 10 stretches.
- Increase the exercise by holding the pose for longer – 20 seconds maximum.

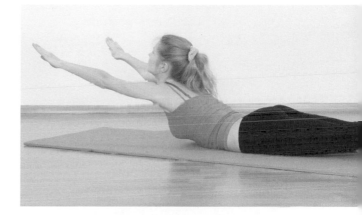

Plank

- Lie face down.
- Bring yourself up and support yourself on both elbows and the tips of your toes.
- Keep your body straight and hold the stomach muscles tight.

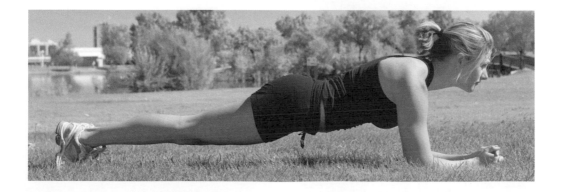

- Hold for 10 seconds.
- Relax for 30 seconds.
- Repeat six times.

- Increase the exercise by holding the pose for longer – 60 seconds maximum.

Side Plank

- Begin in the plank position.
- Roll to the right side so that you are supported only by your right foot and elbow.
- Hold for 10 seconds.
- Relax for 30 seconds.
- Repeat for the left side.
- Repeat for a total of three times on each side.
- Increase the exercise by holding the pose for longer – 60 seconds maximum.

Clams

- Lie on your right side, supporting yourself with the opposite arm.
- Bring both legs up together to 45 degrees.
- Keep the right leg flat on the ground; using your ankles as a 'hinge', raise the left knee.
- Aim to bring the left knee all the way to vertical.
- Lower and repeat slowly 10 times.
- Repeat on the opposite side.
- Complete three sets of 10 on each side.

Joining the Race

Running in an organized race is not the ultimate (or even intermediate) goal for *all* runners. If it's not your idea of fun, then just continue enjoying your training and running purely for its own sake – and the sake of your health. However, with increased confidence and ability, many runners find that they wish to participate in an organized event.

Take Your Pick

With the use of the internet and listings in running magazines, it could not be easier to identify a race to suit you. Make some simple choices about where and when you would like to race (leaving plenty of time for training), pick the type of event and distance you want to run, pay the fee – and you're ready to go!

Be Realistic

Make sure that your race goals are a balance of achievable and challenging. If you can already comfortably run for an hour, aim for a 10k race. Happy running for 90 minutes? Try a 10-miler or even a half-marathon. Push yourself and stay focused.

Keys to Successful Racing

When you've signed up for a race event, there are some top tips to keep in mind to have a successful day.

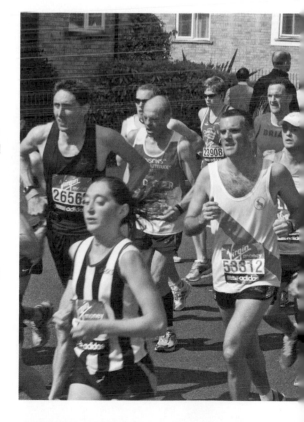

☑ **Arrive early**: Avoid pre-race stress.

☑ **Fuel up**: Make sure you have eaten and drunk adequately before the race.

☑ **Keep it steady**: Aim for a constant speed; do not begin too fast.

☑ **Keep focused**: Concentrate on steady breathing.

☑ **Forget time**: Do *not* worry about your time – this improves with experience.

☑ **Take safety pins**: These are essential for tacking on your race number.

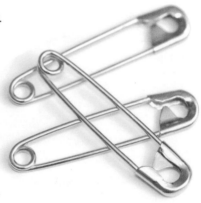

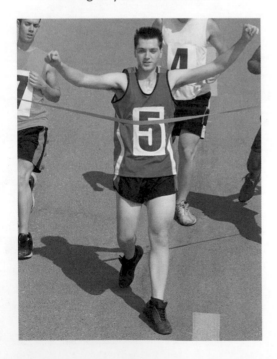

☑ **Stay safe**: Write emergency contact details on the back of your number.

☑ **Follow orders**: Always obey safety instructions and advice.

☑ **Enjoy yourself**: It will all be over (relatively) quickly!

☑ **Cool down**: Walk for five to 10 minutes after finishing.

☑ **Stretch**: Help your muscles recover.

5k Races

There are plenty of short race distances – usually classed as 'fun runs' – but the 5k is probably the first race distance a new runner comes across and considers tackling. If you have followed even the most basic training plans in this book, a 5k race should be well within your capabilities.

Too Fast?

It is worth noting that because of their short distance – although it may not seem short to you yet – 5k races are often much faster and attract a considerable number of club runners aiming for league points and personal-best times. Don't let this put you off! However slowly you intend to run a 5k race, you should always feel just as welcome and valued as the most proficient runner.

Top Tip

If the potential speed of a 5k feels intimidating, consider sticking with your training and pushing straight through to a 10k race. These often attract people with a wider range of ability levels.

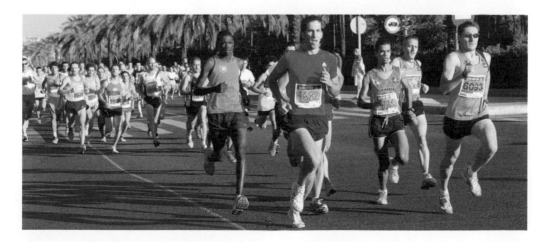

Improving Your 5k Speed

Once you have mastered the distance (*see* page 173), you'll probably want to work on improving your time, and the short, sharp 5k race distance is perfect for goal setting in this. Making small incremental improvements is vital for staying injury free, so do *not* attempt to dramatically increase both speed and distance at the same time.

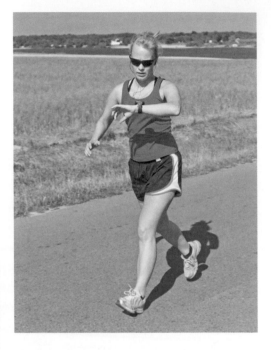

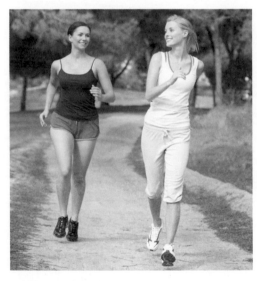

Top Tip

Find a training partner whose pace is just faster than your own. Running with them will slowly draw you up to an equal pace.

Gradual Improvements

Interval and fartlek training (*see* pages 40–42) are both variations on a theme that use repetitions of fast and slow paces over distance to gradually train your body for greater speeds. Both are relatively high-intensity workouts, so they should always be followed with a rest day (or a day of low-impact cross training such as swimming). High-intensity cross training such as a fast cycle ride or a spinning exercise class is an excellent addition to your training when looking to improve speed.

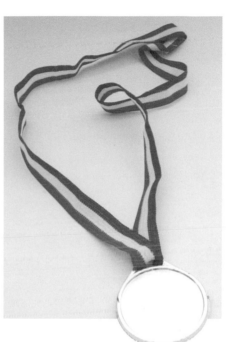

10k Races

There are thousands of 10k races across the country that you can choose from. A popular distance for runners of all abilities, the 10k can present its own challenge in terms of distance or, once you are comfortable with the distance, it can be a great event at which to test your speed.

Mix It Up

10k races take many forms (including both road and trail), but, because they are quite short, many also take a more novel form to increase the challenge. These 'novelty' races may include obstacles, river crossings or

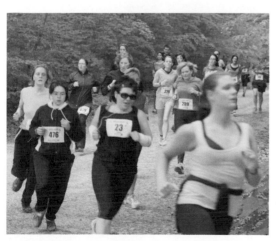

other natural challenges to keep things interesting. Prices vary, but 10ks generally begin at around the £10 mark, making them very affordable. You'll be amazed at how quickly you begin to accrue finishers' medals and other mementos.

As with other distances, running clubs are a great source of information on local races and events. Most clubs also take part in leagues, which cover a series of races in the local area.

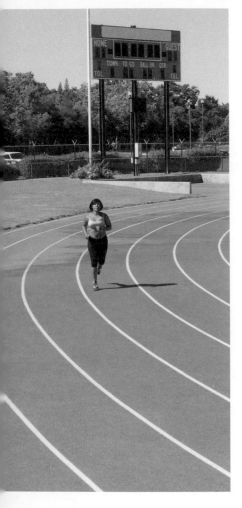

10k Plan

This eight-week plan assumes that you are already capable of running at a steady pace for 35–45 minutes. If you can't, follow the weight loss/health plan on pages 169–72 until you reach this level. Ideally you should have access to a measured 400 m distance (such as a running track). If not, estimate the distance along an unbroken stretch of your usual running route. Following this plan improves speed over a 10k race distance.

Day 1: Run slowly to warm up for five minutes. Run at an easy pace for 3 km. Ten-minute cool-down run and stretch.

Day 2: Run slowly to warm up for five to 10 minutes. Run for 30 minutes at a 'comfortably hard' pace (a speed at which it is just possible to hold a conversation). Ten-minute cool-down run and stretch. This is your 'tempo' run.

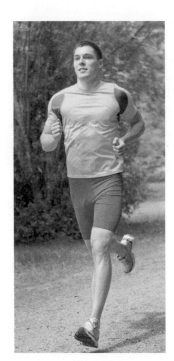

Be Inspired
'Most people race to see who is the fastest. I run to see who has the most guts.'
Steve Prefontaine, running guru

Day 3: Rest.

Day 4: Run slowly to warm up for five minutes. Run at an easy pace for 30 minutes. Ten-minute cool-down run and stretch.

Day 5: Rest.

Day 6: This distance will slowly increase over the weeks up to a maximum of 9 km. Run slowly to warm up for five to 10 minutes, then run 4 km at a gentle pace (below the pace you may wish to race). Ten-minute cool-down run and stretch.

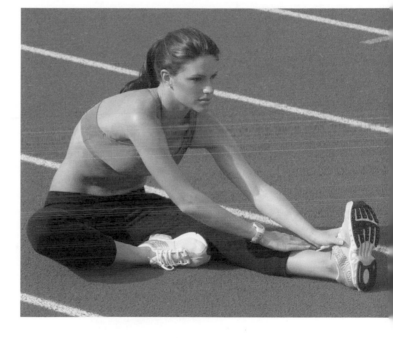

Day 7: Rest.

Week 2: Follow the same routine as week one.

Week 3: Increase day one's easy run to 4 km – keeping it gentle. Increase day two's tempo run to 40 minutes and day six's run to 5 km.

Week 4: Day two now changes to interval training. Run slowly to warm up for five to 10 minutes. Run your measured 400 m at a hard pace, followed by a second 400 m at a very slow run or walk (this is one 'interval'). Repeat the hard pace/slow run 400 m twice more for a total of three intervals. Ten-minute cool-down run and stretch. Increase day six to 6 km.

Week 5: As for week four, but increase day six to 7 km – try running closer to the pace at which you would like to race.

Week 6: Day two's intervals should be increased from three to four repetitions of 400 m hard, 400 m easy. Day six increases to 8 km.

Week 7: Increase day two to five repetitions of 400 m hard/easy. Longest run on day six – 9 km.

Week 8: Rest week leading up to your race on day seven. A very gentle run on day one, two or three – no more than 30 minutes.

Keys to Success

- Always warm up and cool down on each run.
- Do not forget to stretch.
- Drink adequate water before *and* after exercise.
- Rest days are vital for recovery.

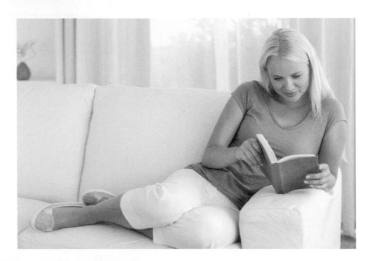

Half-marathon

Half-marathons are one of the most popular and increasingly staged distance runs. With a little dedication and training, this 13.1 mile challenge should be achievable for almost any runner prepared to put in the miles. Almost every city that holds a famed marathon also stages a half-marathon (not always at the same time), which means that if you love the half-marathon, but feel unable to step up to full marathons, you can still enjoy the experience of cheering crowds from London to New York.

A Happy Half-marathon

Here are some top tips for running a successful half-marathon.

 Fuel up:
Make sure you have eaten and drunk adequately before the race.

 Plan ahead:
Check how regularly drinks are provided along the route.

 Be prepared:
Stay well hydrated pre-race.

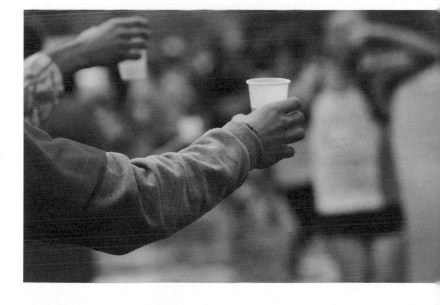

Keep it steady: Start at the same pace you aim to run throughout.

Count down: Mentally tick off each passing mile.

Drink and eat regularly: Fuel your run.

Stick to what you know: Never try new kit, gels or bars on race days.

Set a target time: But stay relaxed about sticking to it.

Top Tip
Ten-mile races are less common, but seek one out as a stepping-stone event between 10k races and your first half-marathon.

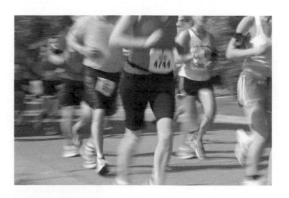

Follow orders: Obey safety instructions and advice.

Cool down: Walk for five to 10 minutes after finishing.

Stretch: Help your muscles recover.

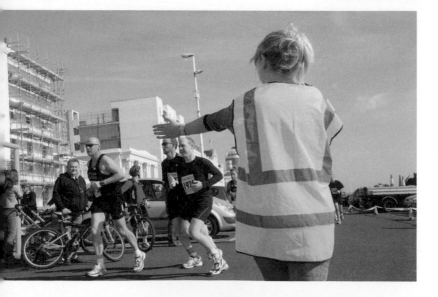

Half-marathon Plan

This 12-week plan assumes that you are already capable of running a 10k race. If not, follow the stamina plan on pages 173–75 first. The key to this plan is gradual increases in the longest run of the week (always on day six), up to a maximum distance of 12 miles – just over one mile short of the half-marathon distance. Do not be tempted to train to the full distance. This plan focuses on achieving the half-marathon distance. If your goal is to improve your time, add a mixture of interval training and fartlek sessions to replace the run on day one of each week. You can also alternate this day with some cross training such as cycling.

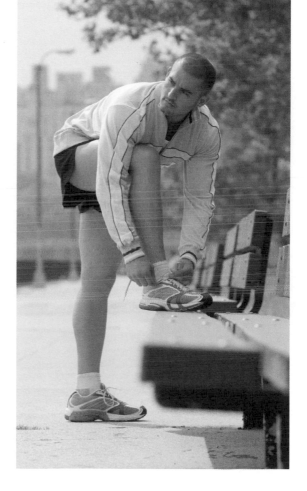

Day 1: Run at an easy pace for 30 minutes. End with a 10-minute cool-down run and stretch.

Day 2: Rest.

Day 3: To build strength (and some speed), this weekly tempo run should be paced just at the upper limit of your comfort zone – a point at which it would be difficult (but not impossible) to hold a conversation. Run slowly to warm up for five to 10 minutes, run at tempo for 30 minutes, 10-minute cool-down run and stretch.

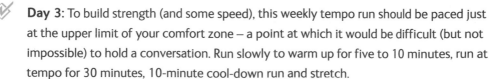

Day 4: Rest.

Day 5: Up until week eight, day five is always the same as day one.

Day 6: Although starting at just three miles, this is the long-run day, which builds each week to the maximum distance of 12 miles (on week nine). Run slowly to warm up for five to 10 minutes. Run at an easy pace for three miles. End with a 10-minute cool-down run and stretch.

Day 7: Rest. This is an increasingly important recovery day as your day six long run increases.

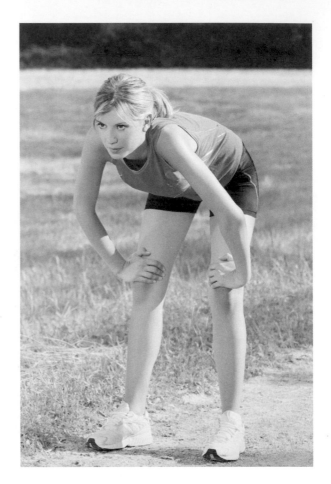

Week 2: The same as week one, but increase day three's tempo run to 40 minutes and day six's distance to 5 miles.

Week 3: Increase day three's tempo run to 45 minutes and day six's distance to 6 miles.

Week 4: Increase day one and day five's runs to 40 minutes each, maintain the 6-mile distance on day six, but try to increase your pace slightly.

Week **5**: Increase the long run on day six to 8 miles. Ensure that you are warming up, cooling down and stretching with each session.

Week **6**: An increase in all times and distances. Day one should be brought up to 45 minutes, day three to 50 minutes and day five to 45 minutes. Push your long run up to 9 miles, focusing on completing your distance without worrying about pace.

Week **7**: Increase day six's long run to 10 miles.

Week **8**: Increase day one and day five to 50 minutes. Increase your tempo run on day three to one hour and your distance on day six to 11 miles.

Week **9**: A *decrease* in the first three runs of the week: Drop day one to 45 minutes, day three to 50 minutes and day five to 40 minutes (no longer mirroring day one). Your longest run of the plan is on day six – this should be 12 miles, keeping a steady pace and remaining focused.

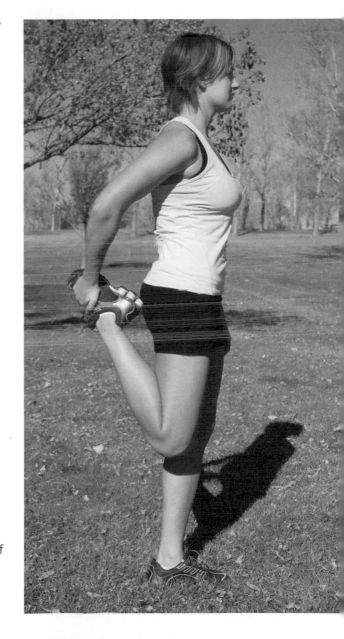

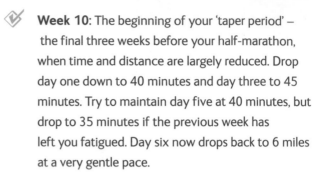

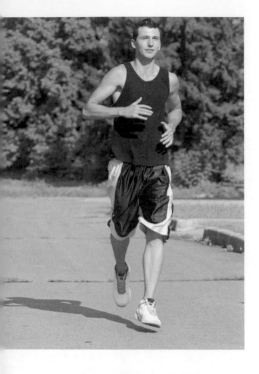

Week 10: The beginning of your 'taper period' – the final three weeks before your half-marathon, when time and distance are largely reduced. Drop day one down to 40 minutes and day three to 45 minutes. Try to maintain day five at 40 minutes, but drop to 35 minutes if the previous week has left you fatigued. Day six now drops back to 6 miles at a very gentle pace.

Week 11: Decrease day one and day five to 30 minutes. Similarly, decrease day three's tempo run to 40 minutes. Continue to aim for 6 miles on day six.

Week 12: Rest week leading up to your race on day seven. A very gentle run on day one, two or three of no more than 30 minutes is okay to include.

Keys to Successful Training

- Follow the plan, but do not panic if you miss a session.
- Keep it varied – replace some of day five's runs with cross training.
- Stay hydrated – water fuels your training.
- Keep nourished, using gels or bars on runs longer than 60–90 minutes.
- Keep a log to record your progress.
- Routine is key – warm up, cool down and stretch.
- Treat any injury immediately.
- Do not over-train – never run further than the recommended 12-mile maximum.

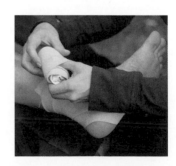

Marathon

For many new runners, the marathon, a gruelling 26.2 miles, is either the ultimate goal or a seemingly unobtainable distance – the reserve of either the elite or the insane. But, as with all running, the secret to undertaking this legendary event is slow, gradual increases in both confidence and ability. As long as you take it step by step, you can achieve that golden distance!

Think It Through

It is often said that a marathon is far more than double a half-marathon and, in all but the most mathematical terms, this is true. Diligently following a training plan might get you through, but mental preparation is equally important. There are times during a race of this length when even the most experienced runners will begin to wilt mentally.

Be Prepared

More than any other distance, carefully studying a race route is crucial; picturing each stage in the mind's eye, and sticking to a strict hydration and nutrition plan will prepare you for the miles ahead. As the old adage has it: 'Plan your run and run your plan.'

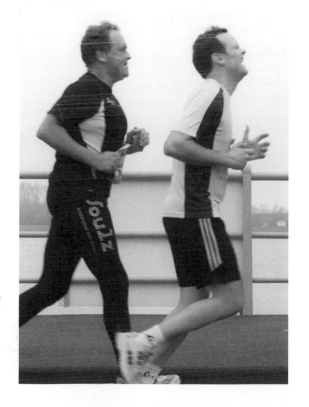

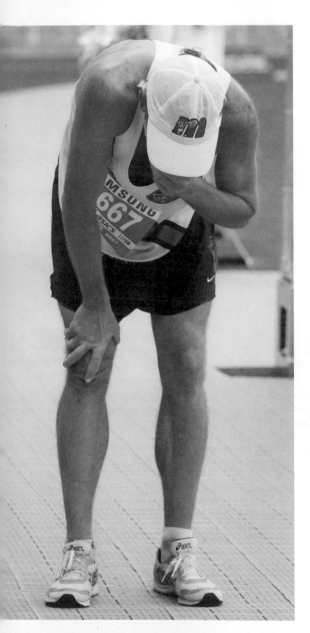

Hitting the Wall

Anyone preparing for their first marathon will have heard about – and undoubtedly feared – 'the wall'. Sometimes this simply refers to the point on the run when you feel both mentally and physically spent, sure that you can't take another step. Technically 'the wall' really means a state of hypoglycaemia, the point at which blood sugars plummet. Careful attention to both pre-race diet, and hydration and nutrition during the race, should help you break through to the other side. The keys to success in a marathon are broadly the same as for a half-marathon (*see page 204*).

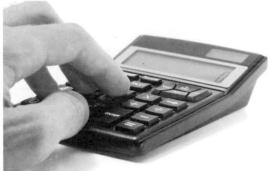

Top Tip
Both half- and full marathons are traditionally marked in imperial miles (as are training plans). To convert to metric, multiply miles by 1.6. A marathon is approximately 42 km.

Marathon Plan

This 16-week plan assumes that you are already capable of running a half-marathon. If you can't, then follow the plan for that distance (*see page 201*).

The key to training for a marathon is to slowly build the longest run of the week until a maximum distance of 22 miles is reached. It is not advisable to include a run of the full 26.2 miles in any training plan, despite the fact that this still leaves an unknown element for race day. Never be tempted to train to the full distance.

This marathon plan also focuses on achieving the distance, rather than improving on speed. If you are looking to increase your pace, add a mixture of interval training and fartlek sessions to replace the base runs which are scheduled for day one of each week in this plan.

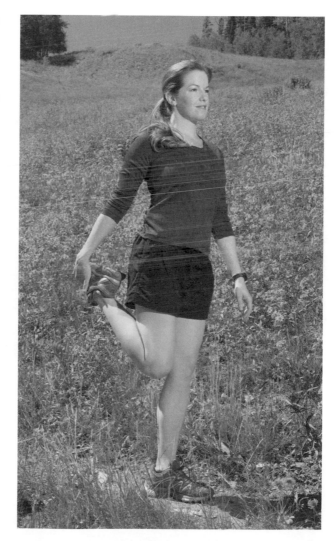

 Day 1: Run slowly to warm up for five minutes. Run at an easy pace for 30 minutes. End with a 10-minute cool-down run and stretch.

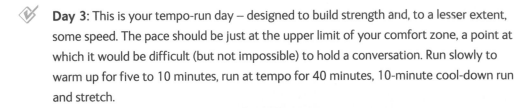

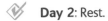 **Day 2**: Rest.

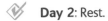 **Day 3**: This is your tempo-run day – designed to build strength and, to a lesser extent, some speed. The pace should be just at the upper limit of your comfort zone, a point at which it would be difficult (but not impossible) to hold a conversation. Run slowly to warm up for five to 10 minutes, run at tempo for 40 minutes, 10-minute cool-down run and stretch.

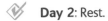 **Day 4**: Rest.

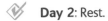 **Day 5**: Up until week 12, day five is always the same as day one. Cross training (such as cycling) can be substituted for a similar duration to bring variety to the training.

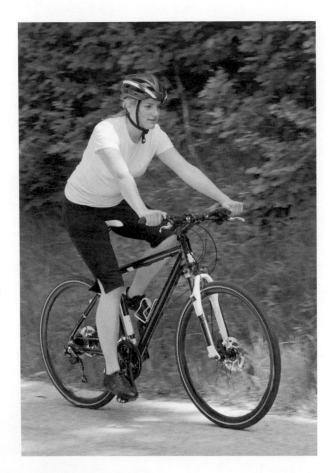

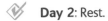 **Day 6**: The long run (but starting relatively short!). Run slowly to warm up for five to 10 minutes. Run at an easy pace for six miles. End with a 10-minute cool-down run and stretch.

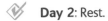 **Day 7**: Rest. This is an increasingly important recovery day as your day-six long run increases.

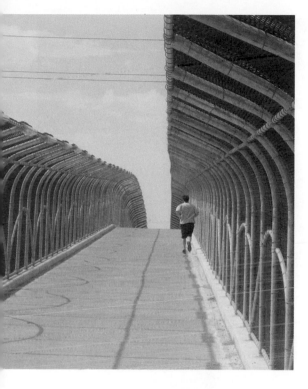

Week 2: As for week one, but increase day six's long run to 8 miles.

Week 3: Increase day three's tempo run to 45 minutes and day six's long run to 9 miles.

Week 4: Increase day one's time to 40 minutes and day five's to 40 minutes. Increase the distance of day six's long run to 10 miles, trying to improve your pace slightly. Continue to observe all the warm-up and cool-down sections of your runs.

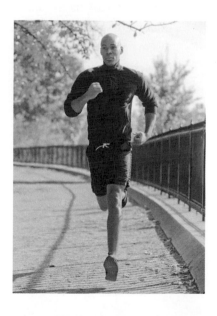

Week 5: As for week four, but increase day three's tempo run to 50 minutes and day six's distance to 12 miles.

Week 6: Repeat week five, but with an increase to 13 miles (almost a half-marathon) on day six.

Week 7: Increase day three's tempo run to 55 minutes and day six's distance to 14 miles.

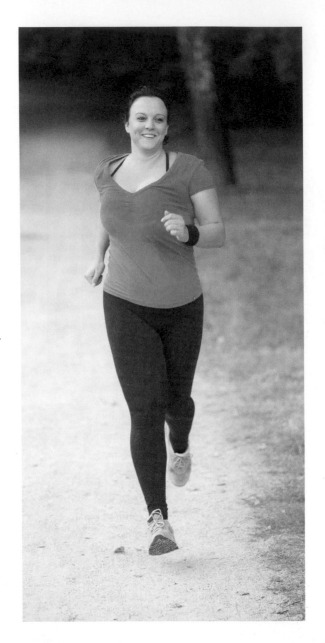

Week 8: An all-round increase. Bring day one up to 50 minutes, day three to 60 minutes, day five to 50 minutes and day six to 15 miles.

Week 9: Day three's tempo run should be *decreased* to 45 minutes, but continue building your long run, bringing day six to 17 miles.

Week 10: This is identical to week nine apart from an increase on day six to 19 miles. Make sure you continue to warm up, cool down and stretch with each run.

Week 11: Bring day three's tempo run back up to 50 minutes and day six's distance up to 20 miles.

Week 12: Increase day one to 60 minutes but *decrease* day five to 40 minutes. Your day-six long run should be brought up to 21 miles.

Week 13: The week of your longest run! All days as in week 12, but push your longest run on day six up to 22 miles. Make full use of day seven's rest.

Week 14: The beginning of your 'taper period', the final weeks before your marathon, when time and distance are reduced in preparation for the big day. Day one is reduced to 40 minutes – keep this very slow, as you are still recovering from week 13's longest run. Day three's tempo run drops to 40 minutes and day five's run to 30 minutes. Day six should be dropped all the way down to a very easy-paced 10 miles.

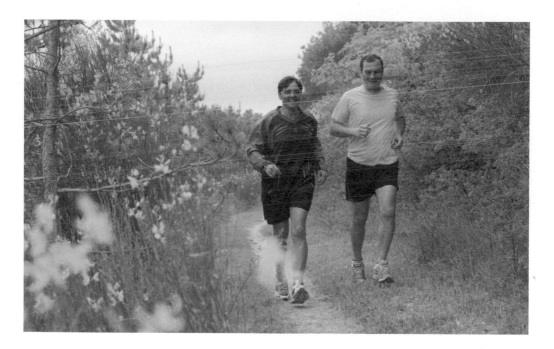

Week 15: Repeat week 14.

Week 16: Rest week leading to race day on day seven. A very gentle run on day one, two or three of no more than 5 miles is okay.

Ultra-running

Extreme distance runs are known as 'ultras', and, whilst technically this applies to anything beyond the standard marathon distance, it is more usually applied to runs in excess of 30 miles.

Be the Best

A number of runners have become true superstars in this area. Chief among them are American Dean Karnazes and Britain's Mimi Anderson, both holders of a range of utterly awe-inspiring world records. Anderson, known as 'Marvellous Mimi', is a grandmother, proving, yet again, that age is no barrier to success with running.

Three of the Toughest

There are several ultra-runs available for the hardiest runners, but the three most difficult are:

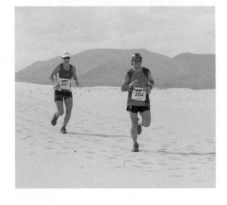

 Marathon des Sables: A six-day, 151-mile (243-km) race across the Sahara Desert in Morocco; competitors must carry everything (except water) they need for the duration.

 Badwater: 135 miles (217 km) of running, without a break, through California's Death Valley to Mount Whitney, in temperatures over 49°C (120°F).

 Spartathlon: Held annually in Greece, this is a 153-mile (246-km) race from Athens to Sparta in celebration of the origins of the modern marathon.

Checklist

✓ **Know your type**: Introvert or extrovert, there is something to be said for both – but keep an open mind about which type of runner you are.

✓ **Keep a log**: There is nothing more motivating than keeping track of the miles you have covered and goals achieved.

✓ **Consider a running club**: Most clubs are friendly and welcoming, so do not be afraid of going along and joining in the fun.

✓ **Follow a good diet**: Never neglect healthy eating when you are training and running hard.

✓ **Check your hydration**: Make sure you drink enough before, during and after training, but also beware of *over-hydration*.

✓ **Follow the guides to successful racing**: From 5k to marathon, there are similar dos and don'ts for each type of race.

✓ **Follow the plan**: Whatever you are training for, try your best to stick to the plan and achieve your goals.

Trouble-
shooting

Injury and Recovery

Is injury an inevitable part of running? Train long enough and hard enough and the answer, regrettably, is probably yes. However, not all injuries are serious and many runners even regard a minor discomfort such as black toenails as a badge of honour. Just listen to competitors before a race, and you'll discover how much more like bragging than complaining their list of injuries is.

Know Yourself

Staying generally healthy, maintaining a good diet and taking a measured and sensible approach to your running and training will drastically reduce the likelihood of any injury. However, accidents do happen and, when an injury does occur, it is important to know how to treat it. If in any doubt about what may be wrong, always speak to a doctor. Similarly, if a condition does not show signs of improvement within the expected time, *always* seek professional advice.

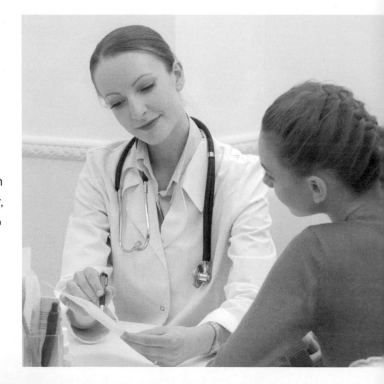

Don't Panic!

Some injuries are inevitable, but these are usually mild – an easily treated blister or a sprained ankle – and seldom career-limiting when it comes to your running. Often when an injury occurs it seems like the end of the world, but once the initial shock and pain have subsided and appropriate measures have been taken to begin the healing process, you'll be amazed at your body's resilience.

Staying Fit When Injured

When it becomes necessary to take a break from running to allow an injury to heal, it is vital to adopt a sensible approach and not push yourself back into running too soon. Equally important is easing yourself back into a running routine following injury – it may feel like starting all over again, but small steps on return from injury will deliver greater long-term gain. Depending on the injury, cycling and swimming are both great ways of maintaining high levels of cardiovascular fitness, and weight and gym sessions can help focus on non-injured muscle groups.

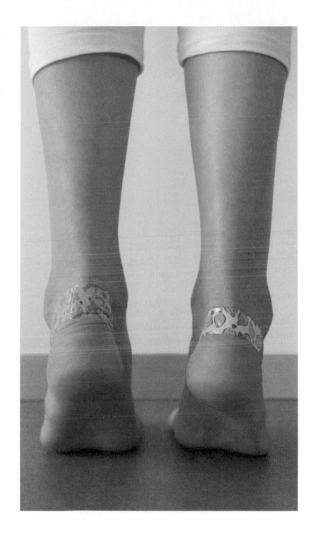

Be Inspired
'Our greatest glory is not in never falling, but in rising every time we fall.'
*Confucius, philosophe*r

Why RICE is Nice

One of the most important concepts for runners is RICE: Rest, Ice, Compression and Elevation. This is the cornerstone of treatment for a huge range of running injuries and ailments. Depending on the nature of your injury, any amount or combination of these four basic elements can set you on the road to recovery.

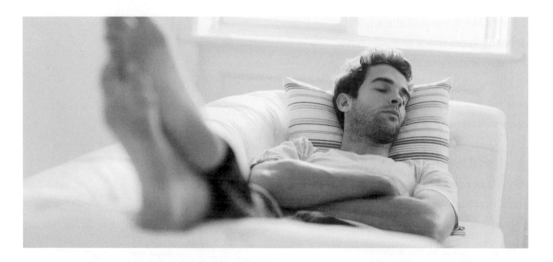

Rest: Depending on the injury, or the severity of the injury, rest can range from a few hours with your feet up to many weeks (even months) away from running. It is vital to listen to your body – and doctor – and take the right amount of time to heal.

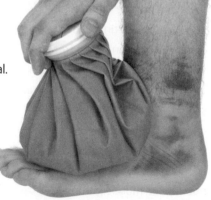

Ice: Many injuries react well (and surprisingly quickly) to the application of ice packs. Cooling an injury as soon as possible will help prevent or reduce swelling, and can also numb any initial pain.

Compression: Compressing an injured area tightly (but not so tightly that blood flow is cut off) will also help to reduce swelling. Apply a bandage, making sure it is clean and sterile, or an elasticated sports support, to help hold the injured area.

 Elevation: Although not always practical, the injured area should be raised above the level of the heart to reduce swelling – so lying on a bed with, for example, the foot supported by several pillows is ideal. You've never had a better excuse for putting your feet up!

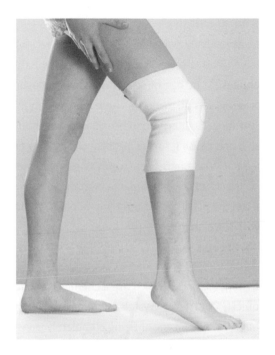

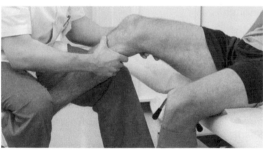

Say 'R'

A sensible variation on RICE is RICER, with the additional R standing for 'Referral to a doctor'. Even experienced runners who are sure they know the nature of their injury and how to treat it are best advised to seek a professional medical opinion.

Getting the Right Temperature

In an emergency, the old-fashioned solution of putting a bag of frozen peas or similar on an injury can do the trick, but there are alternatives that can be used to cool things down and preventing swelling, bruising and pain.

Freezer Solutions

Commercially available ice packs work well, but can have disadvantages. Most importantly (and this applies to the bag of peas too) many domestic freezers can be *too* cold. There is a real danger of suffering 'ice burn' from these packs, damaging the skin and causing further problems. If you do use ice packs or emergency frozen vegetables, make sure that you wrap them in a layer of cloth such as a tea towel and *never* use them in direct contact with the skin.

Quick Packs

Instant ice packs, which use a chemical reaction to quickly cool gel or crystals contained within them, have the advantage of being completely transportable so they can be stored in a kit bag when attending a race or event. On the downside, many are not cold enough to be really effective, and they work only for a short amount of time. Usually they cannot be reused, which makes them a less environmentally friendly option.

Combination Solutions

There are an increasing number of reusable 'coolant bandages' now available, which have several distinct advantages over both traditional and instant ice packs. They combine both the 'I' ('Ice') and 'C' ('Compression') stages of the RICE solution in one – by winding a bandage around the injured area and then spraying it with a coolant spray which draws heat away from the skin to begin the recovery process. Additionally, they provide just the right amount of cooling, and the effect lasts much longer than instant packs.

Be Inspired
'No one ever drowned in sweat.'
***Dan Gable**, wrestler*

Running Injuries

When an injury does strike, it is important to be able to both diagnose it correctly and to begin the appropriate treatment as soon as possible. If you are in any doubt about the nature or cause of an injury, or are concerned that one is not responding to treatment, seek advice from your doctor.

Plantar Fasciitis

This is an inflammation of the thick band of fibrous connective tissue (a bit like a ligament) on the bottom of the foot; it runs from under the heel to the ball of the foot.

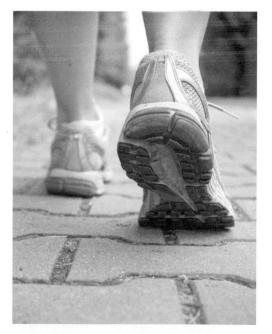

Symptoms

Sometimes a dull ache can be the first sign, after which full-blown plantar fasciitis can develop over several weeks (or runs). The pain is likely to feel worst when you first get out of bed and can vary from a background ache to a sharp pain.

Cause

Badly fitted or brand new shoes can be a cause, but plantar fasciitis is first and foremost an 'over-use injury', most likely to occur if you have recently increased the miles you run. The likelihood of developing it is increased if you overpronate (roll your feet inwards) or fail to warm up before a run.

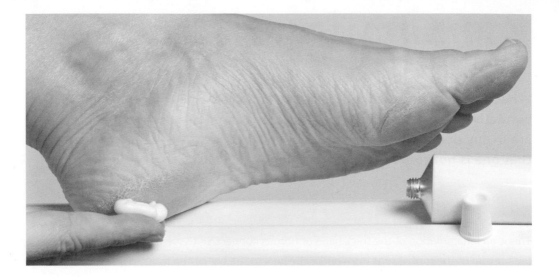

Treatment

An ice pack under the foot will quickly ease the pain, and gentle massage with a foot-roller, combined with the application of a non-medicinal foot cream (peppermint is great), will all speed up healing. The pain will decrease with movement, so many runners continue to exercise more or less as usual.

Heel Bruise

Although not the most serious injury a runner can suffer, a heel bruise can be painful enough to keep you away from training and racing. As the pad of the heel can be thinner in older runners, the chances of suffering a heel bruise increases with age.

Symptoms

The pain can range from mild throbbing to a sharp pain – usually in the middle of the heel pad. It will feel tender when pushed and can be worse when you first get out of bed or if you have been sitting for a long time.

Cause

Insufficient padding through the heel of a running shoe can cause bruising and, as this is often an 'over-use injury', it is more common after particularly long runs – so marathon runners beware! Landing heavily on a sharp stone whilst on the trail can also cause heel bruises.

Treatment

Make sure your running shoes are sufficiently padded and consider well-padded running socks if you find yourself frequently suffering heel bruises. If they develop, use an anti-inflammatory cream and treat with an ice pack. Cushioned heel inserts for shoes (widely available online) can be worn during recovery.

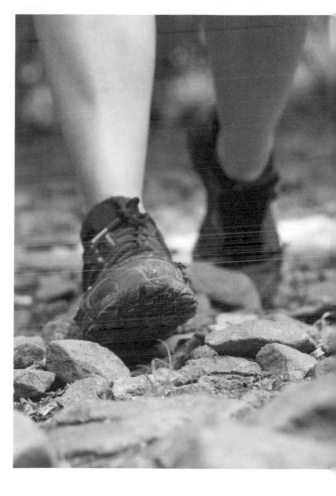

Blisters

Blisters are the body's padding defence (usually against friction), but you are unlikely to feel thankful for this, as few things stop a run faster than a blister. Even a minor 'hot spot' can quickly develop into limping agony.

Symptoms

A feeling of heat and increasing discomfort, most commonly on the heels, toes or around the seams of socks.

Cause

The most common cause is ill-fitting shoes or socks that have become soaked either with sweat or rain.

Treatment

In all cases, prevention is preferable to cure, so make sure that your running shoes are appropriate – always have them fitted and tested by a

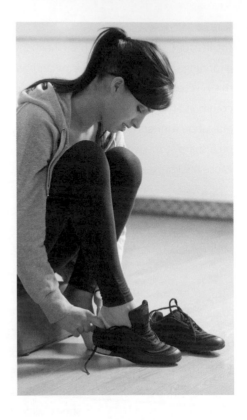

specialist sports shop – and that new pairs are broken in over a series of shorter runs. If you are

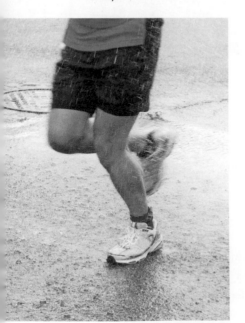

prone to developing blisters, then friction can be reduced using Vaseline or specialist anti-chafing creams. Carry small blister-plasters for rapid treatment on the run; these are much better than regular plasters, as they incorporate a gel padding. Resist the temptation to 'pop' a blister with a pin.

Be Inspired

'To be a good loser is to learn how to win.'
Carl Sandburg, poet

Athlete's Foot

This may seem like a condition you left behind with your schooldays, but this painful fungal infection can strike runners of all ages and is notoriously difficult to cure once established.

Symptoms

Symptoms are most likely to appear either below or between the toes, with cracked and split skin that is painful to the touch, causing general itchiness or irritation.

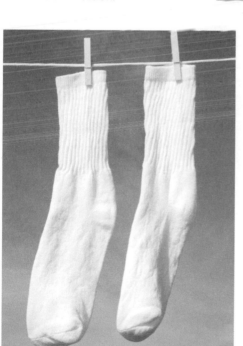

Cause

Athlete's foot is caused by a fungus that thrives in warm, damp conditions. Failing to thoroughly dry your feet after a run, especially if they have been soaked by either rain or sweat, can encourage the fungal infection. It can also be transmitted from others via wet changing-room floors, or even from contaminated soil.

Treatment

Always wear dry, clean socks and make sure that your running shoes are properly dried out before putting them on. Try to avoid too much time barefoot in gym or swimming-pool changing rooms. If athlete's foot does set in, treat it with widely available antifungal creams or powders.

Hard Skin

Thick, hard skin patches can appear on many areas of the foot, but are most common around the heel and ball of the foot. More technically, these patches are known as calluses.

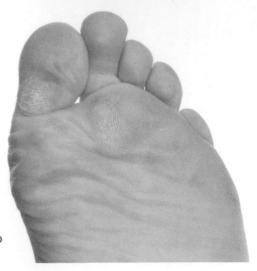

Symptoms

Hard patches on the feet often start small and grow, both in area and thickness – these are not usually painful, but can be yellowish in colour and unsightly. If left untreated, calluses can continue to thicken and affect the fit of your running shoe.

Cause

Calluses are part of the body's natural defence; the skin thickens due to a protective protein called keratin when it experiences rubbing or excessive pressure such as that caused by your running shoes.

Treatment

Use natural pumice to gently rasp away hard skin, then apply a simple foot cream. Pamper your feet once a week with a little moisturizer and ensure your shoes are well fitted.

Cracked Heels

Cracked heels often arise from untreated calluses, and are a common complaint in many runners; initially, they might be just a mild irritation, but they can become infected if left untreated.

Symptoms

A build-up of hard skin around the heel, which can become increasingly uncomfortable. When the hard skin (callus) begins to crack and split, light bleeding can be noticeable and, if this is allowed to develop, infection can set in with swelling and increased pain.

Cause

As with calluses elsewhere on the feet, the build-up of hard skin is usually the body's response to friction, so good socks and well-fitted shoes can help prevention. Runners with drier skin are more likely to develop cracked heels and some medical conditions, including diabetes, psoriasis and eczema, can contribute too.

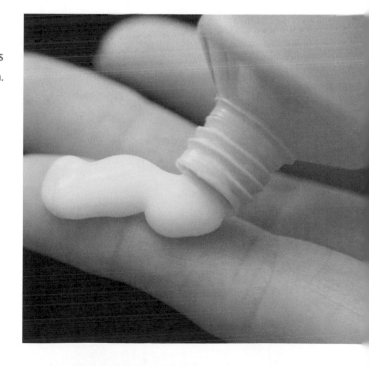

Treatment

Treating patches of skin that are visibly hardening with natural pumice stone and moisturizing creams should prevent the heels from cracking. If the heel has cracked and shows signs of bleeding, treat with an antiseptic cream and take care to avoid infection.

Bursitis

The bursae are tiny sacs of fluid that help reduce friction between bones and tendons or muscles. Although these bursae can become inflamed around a runner's knee, it is also relatively common under the foot and around the Achilles tendon.

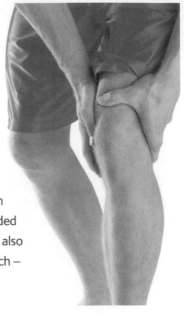

Symptoms

Bursitis in either the knee or underfoot can range from a sharp, sudden pain to a dull background ache or throb. In both cases, the discomfort is often worse after sitting for an extended period (or when you first get out of bed); underfoot bursitis is also likely to hurt more post-run, when it can be tender to the touch – almost like a bruise.

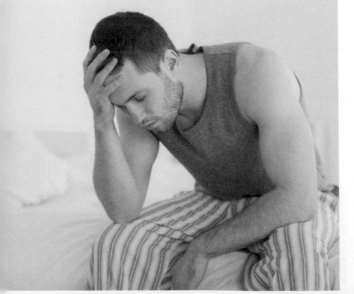

Cause

Bursitis is considered a 'repetition' injury and, as running involves plenty of repetition, it is no surprise that so many runners develop it at some point.

Treatment

Ice packs and over-the-counter anti-inflammatory creams will help, as will taking a break from running. Switching to a more 'giving' running surface when you start training again will ease you back in – try going off-road. More serious bursitis can be treated professionally with steroid injections.

Black Toenails

Black toenails are either the curse of all runners or worn as a badge of honour. Either way, run for long enough and sooner or later you are likely to suffer one or two.

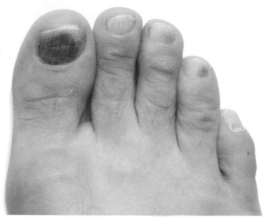

Symptoms

As terrifying as it can look, a black toenail is really just a bloody blister that has developed below the nail, usually along the nail bed.

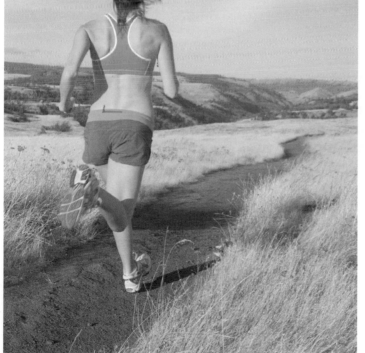

Cause

The most common cause is ill fitting shoes, particularly those that are too big, causing the foot to slide forwards and stub the toes against the inside of the shoe. This usually affects the longest toe, but this is not always the big toe, but rather the second toe next to it. Black toenails are also likely to develop if you do a lot of downhill running, particularly off-road, where the terrain is more punishing.

Treatment

Prevention is better than cure, so make sure that your shoes are well fitted. If you do get a black toenail, you'll probably find that it no longer hurts after a day or two, so is best left alone to heal. Sometimes the nail may fall off as a result of the blister, in which case clean well and treat with antiseptic cream.

Achilles Tendonitis

The Achilles tendon at the back of the ankle attaches the calf muscles of the leg and knee to the heel. It is used when standing on your toes and in the 'pushing-off' part of the stride.

Symptoms

Symptoms are usually pain and inflammation around 4 cm (1.5 in) up from the heel, although the painful spot can be lower. The area will feel tender when pushed gently and there might be a disconcerting 'crackling' feeling beneath the skin. Pain will increase if you stand on tiptoes.

Cause

A sudden increase in training or running can add to the chances of developing Achilles tendonitis, but failing to warm up adequately before a run can also cause it.

Treatment

RICE is the most effective treatment, the 'R' ('Rest') being absolutely crucial – if you continue to run, you may risk a complete rupture of the tendon. Pain around the tendon can be treated with non-steroidal anti-inflammatory drugs, which are available without prescription. A cream version works better than tablets, as the action of rubbing it in works as a gentle massage.

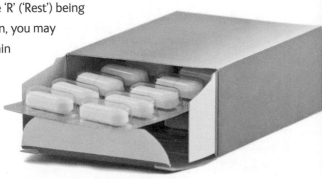

Ankle Sprain

It is estimated that ankle sprains account for about 25 per cent of all sports injuries; all runners are certain to suffer their fair share.

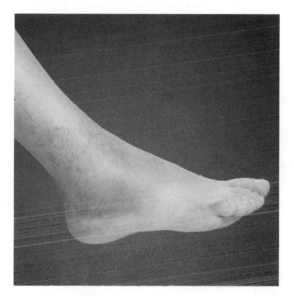

Symptoms

Usually an initial sharp pain in the ankle at the time of injury, followed by a continued dull ache that usually rises to sharp pain when weight is put on the foot. Swelling and bruising can also develop.

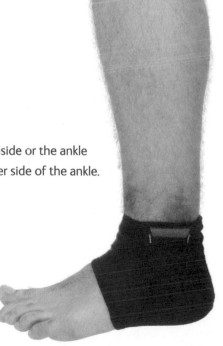

Cause

Most ankle sprains occur when the foot rolls to the inside or the ankle twists, tearing or stretching the ligaments on the outer side of the ankle. Uneven terrain or just a kerb can be responsible.

Treatment

Begin RICE as quickly as possible – an ankle sprain responds brilliantly to this simple self-help treatment. Non-prescription painkillers and anti-inflammatory creams can help, but plenty of rest without the temptation to run is the key.

Stress Fractures

Many runners mistakenly diagnose general aches and pains as stress fractures, but a genuine stress fracture can be a real problem. Some might heal quickly, but others can be truly debilitating.

Symptoms

Most commonly suffered either in the foot (generally the metatarsal bones) or the shins (tibia), sharp pain is usually felt during a run. This will probably increase as the run continues, and may swell and feel tender to the touch post-exercise.

Cause

Badly worn-out shoes or those without adequate padding for your running requirements will add to the chances of suffering a stress fracture. An increase in the distance run, particularly on hard surfaces such as roads or pavements, can result in fatigued muscles that in turn place too much stress on the bones and result in tiny fractures.

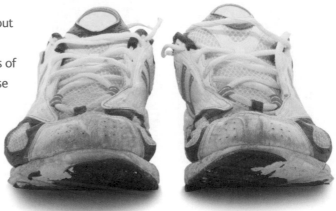

Treatment

Absolute rest is the key to healing – do not be tempted to run *any* distance until fully recovered. When you do begin training again, make sure that the miles are built back up slowly. RICE and anti-inflammatory creams will reduce any swelling and help to manage the pain.

Be Inspired

'I had as many doubts as anyone else. Standing on the starting line, we're all cowards.'
Alberto Salazar, three-time winner of the New York marathon

Shin Splints

Shin splints are one of the most common running injuries, although this might be because the term is often incorrectly used to cover a variety of lower-leg pains. True shin splints are an inflammation of the tendons on the inside of the tibia.

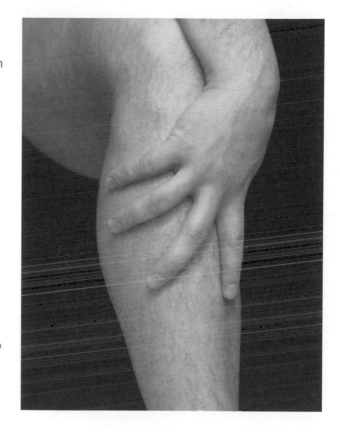

Symptoms

Pain is usually felt radiating out from the midpoint of the shin – about halfway between the ankle and the knee. The throbbing pain usually increases when pressed, but may subside if you continue to run, only to return (probably increased) afterwards.

Cause

Failing to warm up before a run can increase the chances of developing shin splints, as will too much running on hard, unforgiving surfaces – road runners are more likely to suffer than trail runners, though overpronating on any surface makes shin splints more likely.

Treatment

Treat shin splints early with RICE and you will probably nip them in the bud. Continued running will only make things worse and the inflammation will be more problematic to handle. It is vital that frequent sufferers have their running style and shoes carefully checked. An expensive, but sometimes necessary, solution is orthotics – special shoe inserts. A podiatrist can advise on this.

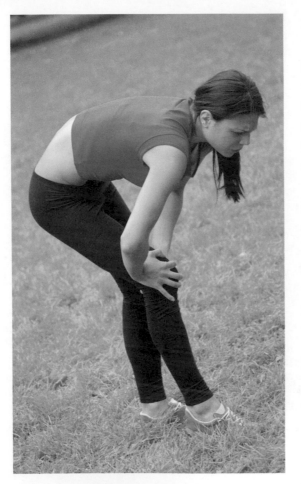

Runner's Knee

The knee is one of the most complex joints directly involved in the motion of running, and is one of the most frequently injured. Although a range of injuries are possible, including damage to ligaments and cartilage, the most common complaint is runner's knee.

Symptoms

Although the term runner's knee is often incorrectly applied to a variety of problems, the true condition is chondromalacia, which causes a sharp pain along the inside of the knee when bent. Swelling can also occur.

Cause

Overpronation and weak quadriceps are the main culprits, but tight hamstrings that have not warmed up to a run can also play a part.

Treatment

RICE is the best treatment – starting the compression and ice as soon as possible with anti-inflammatory cream used to ease the pain and any swelling. Make sure that your shoes are suited to your running style.

Be Inspired

'For me, running is a lifestyle and an art. I'm far more interested in the magic of it than the mechanics.'
Lorraine Moller,
Olympic marathon runner

ITB Syndrome

The iliotibial band (ITB) is a band of thick connective tissue that runs from the hip down the outside of the thigh to a point on the shin just below the knee. Inflammation can lead to ITB syndrome, or ITBS.

Symptoms

Because the inflammation is most common around the knee, this is where you are likely to feel a dull ache, which normally increases on downhill runs. Pain can increase as the run continues, but usually stops immediately afterwards.

Cause

The ITB is thinnest around the knee, so over-use (suddenly increasing your mileage, for example) can rub and cause the inflammation and pain. Overpronators are more likely to suffer ITBS.

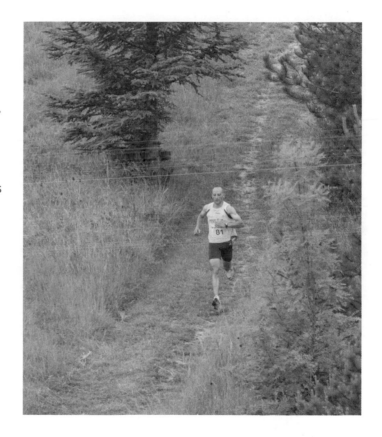

Treatment

RICE starts the healing process, and anti-inflammatory creams should ease any pain — it is a good idea to only slowly begin to increase your mileage again after suffering with ITBS, to prevent its return. A good stretching and warm-up routine can help too.

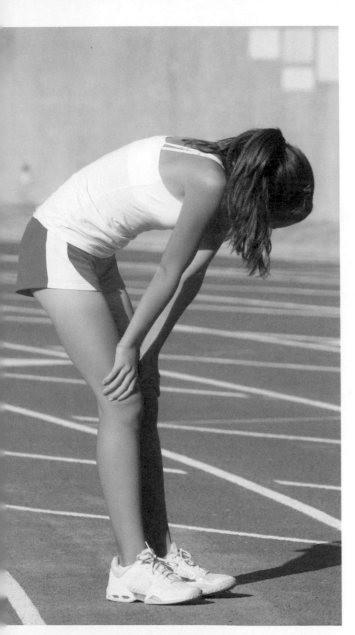

Stitch

A stitch Is something that almost every runner will suffer at some point. The exact cause is still hotly debated, but, whatever it might be, it can stop you in your tracks.

Symptoms

A sharp, stabbing pain is usually felt just below the rib cage or sternum (breast bone). The pain can increase if you try to 'run through it'.

Cause

Most stitches are thought to be caused by a spasm in the diaphragm – the sheet-like muscle at the bottom of the ribcage that functions as part of the breathing process.

Treatment

A stitch will almost always pass completely within a few minutes if you stop running – speed up the process by bending almost double and push with increasing pressure (but not too hard) with your fist below the ribs. It may be possible to halt a stitch whilst still running by exhaling hard in time with the footfall that corresponds with the side that the stitch is on.

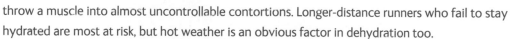

Cramp

A sudden attack of cramp can catch even the most experienced runner off guard, and the sight of competitors at races hopping uncontrollably at the roadside – particularly at long events such as half-marathons and marathons – is a common one.

Symptoms

An extremely sudden 'tight' pain in the affected muscle, which often results in an inability to straighten or flex the area in spasm.

Cause

Dehydration is the most likely cause of a cramp; with dehydration comes a deficiency of body salts, particularly sodium, which can

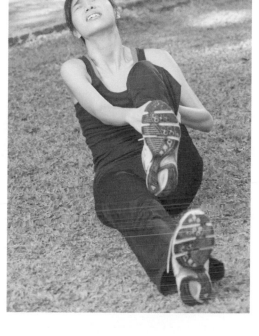

throw a muscle into almost uncontrollable contortions. Longer-distance runners who fail to stay hydrated are most at risk, but hot weather is an obvious factor in dehydration too.

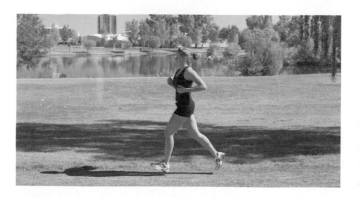

Treatment

Drink appropriately to avoid cramps happening, but, if one does set in, then stopping the run – you are likely to have little choice *but* to stop – and gently stretching and massaging the muscle should quickly loosen things up.

Delayed Onset Muscle Soreness (DOMS)

Along with general fatigue in the days following a particularly long or challenging run, DOMS is almost certain to strike if you don't take proper precautions.

Symptoms

DOMS can range from a general all-over ache to quite highly targeted pains in specific muscles or muscle groups – usually the lower legs (calves) and upper legs (quadriceps, or quads). As the 'D' for 'delayed' suggests, this usually starts 24 or even 48 hours after a run.

Cause

The general pounding from a long run is the overall cause, with everything from microscopic muscle tears to dehydration as contributing factors. Lots of downhill running can cause DOMS of the quads, whilst other factors such as terrain and distance will all play a part.

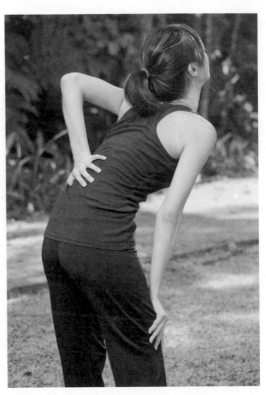

Treatment

RICE and some gentle self-massage, starting from the end of the run and continuing for a day or two, will help reduce the risk of DOMS – as can wearing recovery compression wear (*see* page 89). One of the most common mistakes made by first-time marathon runners is to schedule the next day off work to recover, only to find that it is the day *after that* when things hurt the most.

Be Inspired

'To be number one, you have to train like you're number two.'
Maurice Greene, sprinter

Dehydration

Water is crucial to almost every bodily function, and becoming dehydrated – far more likely in runners because of sweat – can be dangerous to the point of becoming life-threatening.

Symptoms

Cramps, headaches, fatigue and even chills are signs that dehydration is setting in. Perhaps more usefully, your body provides the best warning sign of all: you will feel thirsty. Learn to read the signs, though – it's always best to rehydrate *before* you feel thirsty.

Cause

In runners, the primary cause of dehydration is high temperatures exacerbated by excessive sweating. But beware: dehydration can happen even in cold, cloudy conditions.

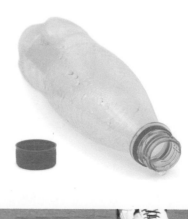

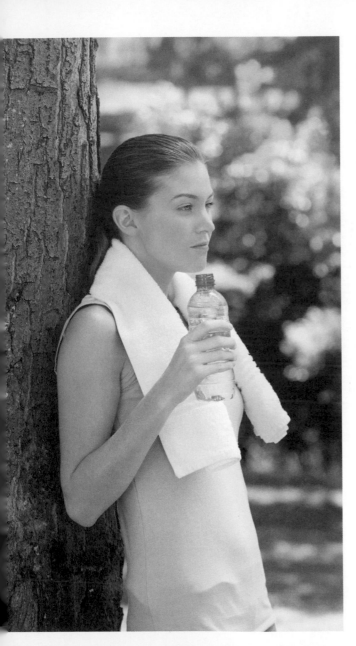

Treatment

*Re*hydration is the simple answer – you will need to start replacing your body's lost water as quickly as possible. Tap water is a start, but, because many of your body's salts will have been lost through sweat, it is advisable to use readily available rehydration tablets. If you feel you are becoming dehydrated on a run, stop immediately, find shade and rest. Never underestimate how serious the condition can be.

Back Pain

Pain in the lower back can have multiple causes, but any chronic or suddenly occurring back pain should *always* be dealt with by a health-care professional – seek advice from your doctor or physiotherapist.

Top Tip

Do not be tempted to head straight for ice-cold water. As refreshing as it might look, very cold water can have an adverse effect on a dehydrated body, causing stomach cramps and nausea.

Symptoms

Symptoms range from low-level aches to more acute pain, from just above the buttocks to around 15 cm (6 in) up the lower back. They are often worse after a hilly run.

Cause

Leg-length discrepancy – one leg being longer than the other, which experts believe affects around a third of the population – is a common culprit for lower-back pain, as is overpronation. Weak core muscles (lower back, side and stomach) can also be a factor.

Top Tip

Use a tennis ball to gently massage the small of the back.

Treatment

Assuming the pain is mild (otherwise, seek medical advice), gentle massage and alternating between ice packs and heat pads – or a hot-water bottle – should help recovery. Anti-inflammatory creams and gels will bring quick relief, but, to avoid the problem in the first place, work on strengthening core muscles (see page 188).

Chafing

Like blisters, chafing might not be considered the most extreme of a runner's injuries, but it can certainly be painful enough to stop you in your tracks.

Symptoms

Chafing symptoms range from small, dry patches of skin to larger areas rubbed almost raw around seams and natural body crevices or between the thighs.

Cause

Friction is the culprit, but this can be caused in one of three main ways: ill-fitting shorts or tops, particularly those with badly designed seams; skin rubbing against skin (between the thighs, underarms and in the groin is most common); or the build-up of sweat.

Treatment

Ensure that shorts and tops are well designed and fitted, and that they can cope with wicking sweat away from the skin efficiently. Keeping well hydrated will also help stop excessive sweat build-up. Although heavier runners may be more prone to chafing around the groin and thighs, almost anyone can suffer – use Vaseline or specially formulated anti-chafing creams before a run and treat any areas that have appeared with either Vaseline or other rehydrating creams. Take care with any particularly raw patches, treating with antiseptic if necessary.

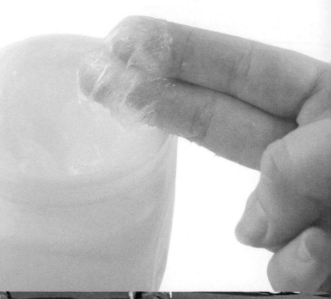

Checklist

✔ **Know your injury**: With experience comes knowledge of injuries. Check with your doctor if you do not know what is wrong.

✔ **Keep an ice pack handy**: So many running injuries respond well to ice that keeping an ice pack permanently on hand is vital.

✔ **Take your time**: Some injuries take longer to heal than others. Bide your time and allow your body to recover.

✔ **Stay fit and focused**: If you are injured, maintain your fitness with crosstraining. Plan your return to running carefully.

✔ **Make a gentle return**: When you are fit enough to resume running, build your distance back up gradually.

✔ **Warm up, cool down and stretch**: Many injuries can be avoided simply by following this advice on *every* run.

✔ **See your doctor**: If your injury is not improving, or you have any other concerns, see your doctor as soon as possible.

Checklists

Included here are the checklists from each chapter. Use them to remind yourself of key points.

Why Run?

☐ **Set your goals:** Even if your targets are initially unfocused – 'to get fit', for example – try to identify goals that will keep you motivated.

☐ **Explore:** Even the most familiar city or suburb takes on a new dimension once you start to run. Seek out the unusual routes.

☐ **Travel more:** Is there somewhere you've always wanted to visit? Chances are there will be a race or running event nearby.

☐ **Get involved:** Either online or off, form a club or get together with others with similar goals and running ambitions.

☐ **Off on holiday?** Pack your running shoes!

☐ **Stay safe:** Online security and safety is vital – keep alert.

☐ **Do it for charity:** What could be more motivating than raising money while you run? Signing up for an event that will push you to train harder too!

☐ **Get eco-friendly:** Seek out events that have a clearly defined environmental policy, or help your local race establish one.

Many Types of Running

☐ **Choose your distance:** Explore the many races, ranging from 5k to marathon (and beyond), listed online. With thousands to choose from, there is certain to be something to inspire.

☐ **Road or trail:** Although it does not have to be a clear-cut choice, most runners start out with a preference, so find out about them and decide which might work for you.

☐ **Choose your kit well:** Road and trail kit (especially shoes) are very different – make sure you have the right gear.

☐ **Is city running for you?** Consider the pros and cons carefully.

☐ **Safety:** Check that your route is safe and take all sensible precautions, especially when training at night.

☐ **Stay hydrated:** Check that you drink enough before and after training. Drink during training too, especially if it is a long or hot session.

☐ **Avoid injury:** Always warm up, cool down and stretch as part of your training routine.

Footwear

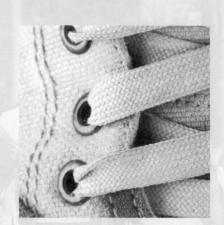

☐ **Trail or road**: Shoes are designed for specific terrains; choose your shoes to fit your routes.

☐ **Check pronation**: Always have a specialist running shop identify your running style.

☐ **Know your type**: Neutral-cushioning, stability, motion-control and performance shoes need to suit your foot's natural design.

☐ **Beware bargains**: Counterfeit shoes are more common than you might think. Always buy from a reputable outlet.

☐ **Multi-terrain running**: Look for trail shoes with low-profile lugs to mix trail and *some* road running.

☐ **Experiment**: Barefoot running is increasingly popular and can improve your running style. It adds variety to your routine too.

☐ **Buying shoes**: Shop in the afternoon; take your time and test *thoroughly*.

☐ **Replace worn shoes**: Nothing causes more injuries than old, badly worn shoes. Check regularly for signs of wear and tear.

Clothing

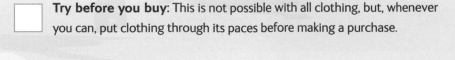

☐ **Check the material:** Running clothing is made from a huge range of materials, but *always* avoid cotton.

☐ **Safety:** Always look for reflectives incorporated into tops, shorts, tights and even socks.

☐ **Stay cool:** Light colours will keep you cooler on a sunny day.

☐ **Seasonal clothing:** Some clothing can be used for both summer and winter, but check suitability before buying.

☐ **Hitting the trails:** Trail running is a specialist area and requires *some* specialist clothing to maximize comfort and enjoyment.

☐ **Check the temperature:** Too hot or too cold and your run will be miserable. Overestimating cold is common, but try to learn from your mistakes.

☐ **Squeeze it:** Compression wear can be expensive, but can bring a range of benefits for both improving performance *and* speeding recovery.

☐ **Try before you buy:** This is not possible with all clothing, but, whenever you can, put clothing through its paces before making a purchase.

Gadgets

☐ **Need vs. want:** How worthwhile is the latest gadget? Make sure your money is well spent and avoid buying something that just looks good.

☐ **Check the evidence:** What scientific proof does the latest gizmo offer for improving your running or health?

☐ **Count the cost:** If all you want to know is how far you have run, a simple pedometer might win out over an expensive GPS device.

☐ **GPS needs:** Check which goals you have set. Which additional GPS features will measure your improvements or aid your training?

☐ **Safety:** How much safety kit do you have? There is no such thing as too much visibility.

☐ **Get in the zone:** Do you need to measure your heart rate? If you want to work 'in the zone', an HRM is essential.

☐ **Sound advice:** Is your route safe for listening to music?

☐ **Stay hydrated:** Make sure you can safely and comfortably carry enough water for a run. Consider the wide range of hydration solutions carefully.

☐ **Pack fit:** From bum bags to full race packs, make sure you can comfortably carry all your food and water, but never overload yourself when setting off for a run.

Getting Started

☐ **Check your fitness**: Take time to get some base measurements, such as blood pressure, weight and heart rate. This gives you a starting point against which to measure your progress.

☐ **Take the first steps**: Take things slowly – never be afraid to drop your pace and walk. Becoming a runner takes time and patience.

☐ **Safety**: Check that your route is safe and take all sensible precautions, especially when running at night.

☐ **Watch what you eat**: Pay careful attention to your diet, read food labels and listen to your body's needs.

☐ **Stay hydrated**: Check that you are drinking enough before, during and after running.

☐ **Identify your goals**: Look at your reasons for wanting to run. This makes it far easier to measure your progress.

☐ **Avoid injury**: Always warm up, cool down and stretch as part of your running routine.

☐ **Mix it up**: Cross training adds variety and helps to build all aspects of training. Make it fun.

Training and Advanced Running

☐ **Know your type:** Introvert or extrovert, there is something to be said for both – but keep an open mind about which type of runner you are.

☐ **Keep a log:** There is nothing more motivating than keeping track of the miles you have covered and goals achieved.

☐ **Consider a running club:** Most clubs are friendly and welcoming, so do not be afraid of going along and joining in the fun.

☐ **Follow a good diet:** Never neglect healthy eating when you are training and running hard.

☐ **Check your hydration:** Make sure you drink enough before, during and after training, but also beware of *over-hydration*.

☐ **Follow the guides to successful racing:** From 5k to marathon, there are similar dos and don'ts for each type of race.

☐ **Follow the plan:** Whatever you are training for, try your best to stick to the plan and achieve your goals.

Troubleshooting

☐ **Know your injury**: With experience comes knowledge of injuries. Check with your doctor if you do not know what is wrong.

☐ **Keep an ice pack handy**: So many running injuries respond well to ice that keeping an ice pack permanently on hand is vital.

☐ **Take your time**: Some injuries take longer to heal than others. Bide your time and allow your body to recover.

☐ **Stay fit and focused**: If you are injured, maintain your fitness with crosstraining. Plan your return to running carefully.

☐ **Make a gentle return**: When you are fit enough to resume running, build your distance back up gradually.

☐ **Warm up, cool down and stretch**: Many injuries can be avoided simply by following this advice on *every* run.

☐ **See your doctor**: If your injury is not improving, or you have any other concerns, see your doctor as soon as possible.

Further Reading

Bannister, Roger, *The First Four Minutes*, The History Press Ltd, 2004

Bolt, Usain, *Usain Bolt: 9.58*, HarperSport, 2010

Coates, Paula, *Running Repairs: A Runner's Guide to Keeping Injury Free*, A&C Black Publishers Ltd, 2007

Coe, Sebastian, *Better Training for Distance Runners*, Human Kinetics Publishers, 1997

Denison, Jim, *The Greatest: The Haile Gebrselassie Story*, Breakaway Books, 2004

Glover, Robert, *The Competitive Runner's Handbook*, Penguin, 1999

Gotaas, Thor, *Running: A Global History*, Reaktion Books, 2009

Harvie, Robin, *Why We Run*, John Murray, 2011

Holmes, Kelly, *Kelly Holmes: Black, White & Gold - My Autobiography*, Virgin Books, 2008

Jones, Bill, *The Ghost Runner: The Tragedy of the Man They Couldn't Stop*, Mainstream Publishing, 2011

Karnazes, Dean, *Ultramarathon Man: Confessions of an All-Night Runner*, Jeremy P. Tarcher, 2006

Karnazes, Dean, *50/50: Secrets I Learned Running 50 Marathons*, Grand Central Publishing, 2009

Kowalchik, Claire, *The Complete Book of Running for Women*, Simon & Schuster, 1999

McDougall, Christopher, *Born to Run: The Hidden Tribe, the Ultra-Runners, and the Greatest Race the World Has Never Seen*, Profile Books, 2010

Murakami, Haruki, *What I Talk About When I Talk About Running*, Vintage, 2009

Noakes, Tim, *Lore of Running*, Human Kinetics Europe Ltd, 2002

Radcliffe, Paula, *Paula: My Story So Far*, Pocket Books, 2005

Stroud, Mike, *Survival of the Fittest: The Anatomy of Peak Physical Performance*, Yellow Jersey, 2004

Swale Pope, Rosie, *Just a Little Run Around the World*, HarperTrue, 2009

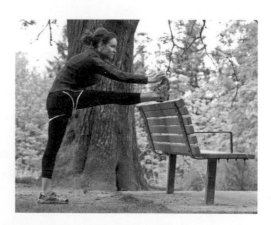

Websites

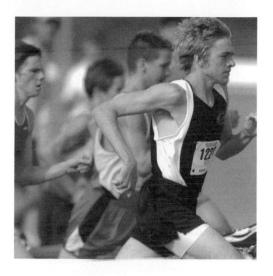

www.bupa.co.uk/running
An excellent range of training plans for 5k, 10k,
10-mile, half-marathon and marathon, with options
on each for a range of abilities — all supported by a
host of tips and features.

www.coolrunning.com
Running news from around the world, plus event
results and features ranging from nutrition to training.

www.fetcheveryone.com
The ultimate online running community. Free to
register and use for logging runs, sharing routes and
discussing topics across every area of the sport.

www.healthynutritionguide.info
A no-nonsense website with all the basics on nutrition to
help you tell your molybdenum from your magnesium.

www.livestrong.com
Although not specific to running, this site is one of
the best resources on the web for health, fitness,
training and far more besides.

www.marvellousmimi.com
Mimi Anderson is one of the most inspirational people
(let alone runners) in the world. Her charming website
leaves mere mortals wondering how she does it.

www.runbritain.com
Focused firmly on road running; despite its name, this
site offers an excellent range of videos that will
appeal regardless of which country you run in.

www.runnersworld.co.uk
The website for this popular running magazine is
packed with free features, tips, training advice,
forums and comprehensive race listings.

www.running4women.com
Free registration for access to a wealth of running
knowledge tailored specifically for women.

www.runningmonkey.co.uk
Dedicated to ultra-distance running, with features,
kit reviews and a list of the world's toughest races.

www.runningpast.com
Detailed essays on the history of running and many
of the sport's greatest champions, plus memorabilia
and autographs.

www.therunningbug.co.uk
All the usual running and training features, but with
an excellent slant on comprehensive forums.

Index